RA

NANCY CAIN

HEALING

THE CHILD

A MOTHER'S STORY

An Inspirational & Practical Guide

for Parents When Kids Are Sick

RAWSON ASSOCIATES

Rawson Associates
Scribner
Simon & Schuster Inc.
1230 Avenue of the Americas
New York, NY 10020

Designed by SONGHEE KIM
Set in Goudy Old Style

Manufactured in the United States of America

10 9 8 7 6 5 4 3 2 1

Library of Congress Cataloging-in-Publication Data
Cain, Nancy Woodard.
Healing the child : a mother's story : an inspirational
& practical guide for parents when kids are sick / Nancy Cain.
p.   cm.
1. Sick children—Care.   I. Title.
RJ61.C16 1996   96-3568
649.8—dc20   CIP
ISBN 0-684-80169-8

To Marty, who someday will understand;
and to my mother, who taught me the importance of faith

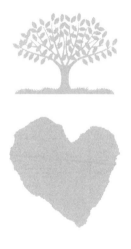

ACKNOWLEDGMENTS

Writing this book has rekindled memories of some of the worst moments of my life. But in those memories are recollections of some of the finest people I have ever met—compassionate people who performed exceptionally kind and unselfish acts. Although it is difficult to list the names of everyone who contributed to the ideas, feelings, and spirit of this book, many of them deserve special mention:

My husband, Tom, deserves the greatest thanks. He's the best companion, friend, father, and editor anyone could ever have.

I feel very fortunate through writing this book to have met my agent, Connie Clausen. It was she who introduced me to another amazing woman, Eleanor Rawson, my editor. These two women gave me a whirlwind education and have truly been an inspiration to me as a writer.

Acknowledgments

Special thanks go to the entire staff of the Medical ICU of Children's Hospital in Boston, and particularly to Jennifer Berkman, Lou Ann Brancato, Mairead Desmond, Jed Gorlin, Patricia Kent, Michael McManus, and John Yee, whose loving care for Alex contributed to many of the ideas I present in this book. Thanks also go to the entire staff of the 9 East pediatric floor, and especially to Jill Driscoll, Suzanne Gracca, and Suzanne Kavet. We will also always remember the Clement family and the Sullivan family, who, as other parents undergoing similar situations with their children, gave us the courage to keep fighting for Alex.

Alex wouldn't be alive today if not for the team effort of many people at Deerfield Valley Rescue in Wilmington, Vermont; Brattleboro Memorial Hospital; and Children's Hospital at Dartmouth Medical Center. From them we learned a lot about volunteerism, guts, and the determination to keep going despite the odds. I would like to give special mention to Ted Newcomb, Karen Moreau, Jim Filiano, David Moody, and Carolyn Strohbehn.

I would also like to thank Cheri and Martin Woodard, Lynn Jelinski, Ted and Betsy Newcomb, Maribeth Ortega, Karen Moreau, Mary Margaret Cain, and Marie Woodard for their helpful suggestions and comments on earlier versions of the manuscript.

Jo Yoder and Maureen Mitchell of Parent to Parent of Vermont were excellent sources of research material on assistance for ill, injured, and disabled children. Jeanne Walsh, the librarian of Dover Free Library, did a great job as usual of locating hard-to-find materials.

And for all the other people we met along Alex's journey to recovery, a big thank-you. More than anything else, you taught us about the incredible healing power of people who care.

Contents

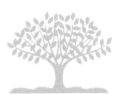

Contents

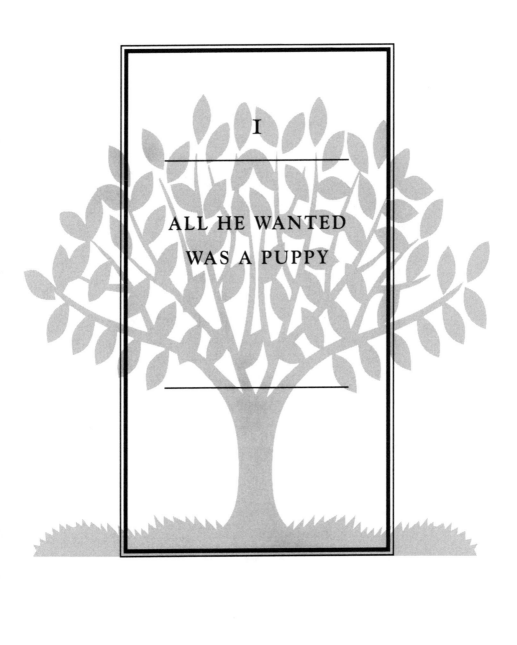

I

ALL HE WANTED
WAS A PUPPY

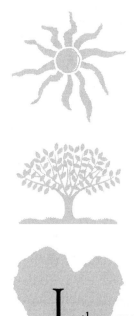

In the summer of 1993, my four-year-old son, Alex, contracted a deadly *E. coli* bacterial infection known as the "Jack in the Box" illness. He didn't eat at a fast-food restaurant. He didn't even eat meat. He wasn't knowingly in contact with anyone else with the infection. In fact, his was the only case that summer in the entire state of Vermont. In the space of forty-eight hours, he went from a healthy child to a child near death.

It was Alex's fourth birthday. My mother had come from South Carolina for his birthday, and we had decided to make it a small family reunion. My brother and his wife had flown in from Virginia for the occasion. My sister and her husband had arrived from up-state New York. It was a perfectly clear, breezy summer day at our mountaintop home, and everyone was gathered on the back deck to catch up on a year's worth of family news. Upstairs, I sat on our bed with Alex, listening to the laughter drift up through the open window overlooking the deck. Despite the fact that family had come a long way to see him, Alex said his stomach hurt, and he wanted to be alone. Too much cake at his preschool birthday party earlier in the day, we thought. We postponed his birthday celebration that evening because he wasn't feeling well enough to eat.

The next day he was worse. When he started passing bloody diarrhea, we became alarmed and called the pediatrician. Preliminary blood work indicated that he had a bacterial infection. No one dreamed at the time that he had the same bacteria that sickened hundreds and killed three children three thousand miles away in Washington State earlier in the year. He was put on an antibiotic, and a stool sample was sent off for a culture. A day went by, and his condition didn't improve. He grew so weak he couldn't hold his head up, and we had to spoon fluids down his throat to get him to drink. Constantly in contact with the pediatrician, my husband, Tom, and I kept asking when the antibiotic was going to work.

I was up most of the night with him. At 2:30 A.M. Sunday morning, he woke up screaming in pain with more diarrhea. I cleaned him up, and rubbed his back to calm him down. After a long while, he fell back to sleep. I finally fell asleep myself next to him, only to be awakened at 4:00 A.M. by the bed shaking—he was locked in a fetal position, having an uncontrollable seizure. It took the ambulance forty-five minutes to wind up the dirt roads to our house and another forty-five minutes to get to the country hospital in Brattleboro. Our two-and-a-half-year-old son, Marty, woke up just as the ambulance was pulling away. He was crying hysterically when I handed him to my visiting mother, telling her to take care of him, to give him whatever he needed. She later told me he spent the entire morning opening and shutting the back doors of his Matchbox ambulance, trying to comprehend what had happened to his brother.

Our pediatrician met us at the emergency room. She immediately recognized the severity of Alex's condition and sent for a pediatric transport ambulance to take him to Dartmouth-Hitchcock Medical

Center. We weren't allowed to see our son as they worked on him, but it seemed like the entire night staff was summoned behind the curtain. Through the muffled voices we could detect a sense of urgency that bordered on panic. Outside the glass doors, we sat arm in arm on the cold cement of the ambulance dock and numbly waited.

It was nearly two hours before our pediatrician came out to update us on his condition. She was wearing the jeans she had hastily thrown on at 5:00 A.M. Her hair was disheveled, she was sweating, and she made no attempt to conceal her anxiety. She told us the lab had just called with news that the stool culture was positive for *E. coli* 0157:H7, the killer "Jack in the Box" bacteria. Did we know what that meant? We knew our son was very sick, but up until that point, we never thought he might die. All she could do was hug us and say she was sorry. I called my mother, who agreed to stay a few days longer to care for Marty. My sister, who had just arrived at her own home, turned around and drove five hours back to help my mother out.

It took a long time to stabilize Alex before he was loaded in the pediatric transport unit and driven sixty miles to the regional medical center. His blood pressure and red cell count dropped dramatically and his belly filled up with fluid. We were asked for permission to give him a transfusion. I naively insisted that I wanted him to have *my* blood, and I was ready to donate it on the spot. Little did I know that over the next week of his life he would require the blood products of 140 different donors.

He was operated on immediately upon arrival. A large section of dead bowel was removed and a colostomy was performed. His condition was so unstable that the surgeon had to leave the wound open for the night. No one was even guardedly optimistic. The surgeon told us to prepare for the likelihood that he might die. Meanwhile, the bacteria that had killed his bowel was continuing its march through his body attacking every organ in its path. We were relieved that he made it through the night, but disheartened to find out in the morning that no antibiotic could stop the bacteria—it was going to have to run its course.

When I came back to the house alone the next day, I saw his scuffed Nike sneakers perched on the stairs. I automatically opened a nearby dresser drawer and shoved them out of sight. My mind flashed back to 4:00 A.M. the morning before when they slid him into the ambulance and swept the doors shut. I knew I couldn't come home again and see those empty sneakers. Worse yet, I couldn't bear the thought that he might never wear them again. I dropped down on the steps, dizzy from emotional exhaustion and sobbed until every muscle in my body hurt.

I drove the two hours back to the hospital filled with fear, anger, grief, and helplessness. I reached the hospital, relieved that I was finally there, but dreading what I might find. Tom's pale, drawn face and sunken eyes were all the update I needed. Nothing had changed. Alex lay comatose, colorless, chugging away on the respirator. There were so many lines and tubes coming to and from his body that I had to hold his big toe—it was all I could hug. In the darkened intensive care unit that night we sat beside him, talked to him, and tried to give him hope. The only answer was the hissing of the respirator, the pulsing tone of the oximeter, and the cacophony of alarms, blurps, and beeps throughout the unit.

That night, Tom cried for the first time in seventeen years. "He always wanted a dog," he said, "and I kept telling him he couldn't have one until he was older. That's all he really wanted." We cried together for a long time. Tom promised to get my son a puppy if he recovered, and that puppy became our symbol of hope. Again and again we told Alex we loved him and to keep fighting because Daddy was *finally* going to give in and get him a dog.

For two days he lay comatose in the pediatric intensive care unit of the regional medical center. Then his kidneys failed, and he had to be transferred to a children's hospital for dialysis. It took an entire day to stabilize his condition enough to make the trip by ambulance 150 miles away. We drove separately by car, not knowing whether we were going to Boston to claim his body or to continue with his treatment. It was nearly midnight, it was raining lightly, and a dense fog made it almost impossible to navigate through an unfamiliar city. We arrived weary from lack of sleep and rattled by our journey. We were met by two critical care physicians who told us very directly that Alex's prognosis was quite poor—only one out of thirteen children this sick with the same illness had survived. The anger that had been building in me over the past two days finally exploded, and I interrogated them mercilessly for two hours. In the end, we became a team. None of us was going to give up without a fight.

When we were allowed in to see Alex, I had a hard time believing it was him. His body had nearly doubled its size with fluid retention. At first I thought he had lost great quantities of hair. Then I realized he was so swollen that his full head of hair was reduced to a little toupee. I held his hand, which felt like a warm water balloon, next to my face and wondered if I would ever get my son back. The toxin produced by the *E. coli* bacteria was producing the typical paradoxical reaction in Alex. At the same time it was cutting off the blood supply to each of his organs, it was also causing uncontrollable bleeding at his surgical site. It was a constant battle to maintain his blood pressure.

We made it very clear to the attending physicians and residents that we wanted everything possible done for our son as long as there was any hope that he was neurologically intact. They told us they couldn't do an EEG or a CAT scan to assess brain function until he was off the respirator, which would be in about three weeks. "Not acceptable," we said. "We *have* to know what we are saving." The next day, his second day in Boston, they did an EEG. Despite the vibrations of the respirator, they were able to detect brain wave activity. We continued aggressively with his treatment.

Our careers as writers allowed us to put our lives on hold so that we could stay at Alex's side. We took turns sitting at his bedside. We talked to him, we told him silly stories, and we read to him. Sometimes we were so physically and emotionally exhausted that we just held on to him and dozed in a rocking chair beside his bed.

We quizzed the nurses on every detail of his care and questioned every specialist who visited him. We asked for reading material on his illness, and we talked openly with his medical team. One minute his vital signs would be stable, then suddenly his blood pressure would sink. They would start another blood transfusion, and the cycle would repeat itself again.

In the afternoon of Alex's second day in Boston, our pediatrician drove three hours to visit him and to give us a pep talk, but even she acknowledged that he might not live. Tom and I began to talk more openly about the effect Alex's death would have on our lives. But around him, we remained upbeat and positive. We put up a picture of him at his bedside and placed his favorite stuffed toy next to his cheek. Both nurses and residents joined in, urging him to get better so that he could get his puppy. For the next three days, we defined the future in one-hour increments.

At night we slept on a cot in the communal parents' room just outside the critical care unit. It was during that time that Tom took to sleeping with Alex's old baby blanket nestled by his head. At 5:00 A.M. on the sixth day, the phone in the parents' room rang, and we knew it was for us. The night before, Alex's blood pressure had begun another downward slide. We had gone into the parents' room at 10:00 P.M. to sleep, unable to take the increasing level of stress at his bedside. As if things weren't unreal enough, that night I had an extraordinary dream. I saw a black screen. Across the top left part of the screen a tiny winged creature that clearly resembled Alex fluttered. Then it turned into a white, luminous butterfly, flew up, and disappeared.

We threw on our clothes and raced into the critical care unit. A crowd of people encircled Alex's bed. The same residents were there from the night before. It had been a long night—their eyes were bloodshot and some clearly needed a shave. The team leader took us aside and informed us that Alex's blood pressure had continued to slide during the night, despite continuous blood transfusions and maximum amounts of medication. They suspected he was bleeding uncontrollably in his gut, and perhaps in his head. There was nothing more they could do, and the end was near. The crowd retreated so that we could be alone with him for the last time. I went in, held his hand, and told him he had been a fighter to the end. I couldn't bear to stay more than a moment. My husband went in and later told me he couldn't bring himself to say what he wanted, "I'm going to miss you, guy." Instead, he simply kissed his forehead.

We sat together in a darkened conference room and cried and cried. I called my family, who had all returned to Vermont given the gravity of Alex's illness. Even my youngest brother and his wife had flown in from Chicago. It was 6:00 A.M., and I woke up my mother. She later told me that I awakened her from a dream in which she was taking Alex by the hand down a long dark tunnel to the outstretched hands of a tall man dressed in black. Just outside the tunnel was her mother, who had died seven months earlier. She let out a long moan when I told her Alex wasn't going to make it. She could hardly talk, but managed to get out that my entire family was there for us. I hung up the phone, and we waited.

Suddenly, there was a knock on the door, and one of Alex's physicians came in. Something inexplicable had occurred. The uncontrollable bleeding had abruptly stopped, and a huge blood clot had formed at his surgical site. His blood pressure had begun to stabilize. Alex had refused to give up. For the next seventy-two hours, Alex's condition improved, although he remained in a coma. His steadfast will to survive so amazed his medical team that he was nicknamed "the Miracle Child." He had made it through a near-death experience, but his illness was hardly over.

Blood levels indicated that the bacteria's toxin had run its course. The big question now was, what had we saved? We were insistent that a CAT scan be done as soon as possible. Couldn't they figure out a way to do a CAT scan even though he was still on the respirator? (The problem was that metallic parts of the breathing apparatus would interfere with the scan, which was based on

X rays.) They agreed to rig up a system to manually breathe for him so that the CAT scan could be done the next day.

That night, at 2:00 A.M., there was a knock on our door. We panicked, but the news was good. The night nurse informed us that Alex was semiconscious and had indicated he wanted to see us by a slight nod of his head. We rushed to his bedside, but he had fallen back into the coma. Maybe she had imagined it. The next morning, he was semiconscious again. I asked him several times to wiggle his toes (his only body part free of some tube or line). No response. "Come on, big guy," I said. "Get those piggies moving!" First a jerk, then a wiggle, and I burst out crying. I remembered the magic of his first smile at five weeks of age. Seeing him wiggle his toes in response to my voice was a hundred times more powerful. The news from his CAT scan was good—there were no obvious signs of permanent damage.

Once the immediate crisis had passed, we decided it was time to bring the family back together. Almost ten days had passed, and my mother and sister needed to return to their lives and careers. They brought Marty to Boston and left him with us. He arrived with one suitcase full of clothes and another full of stuffed animals that he had come to rely on for comfort. For several days, we did not take him in to see his brother because Alex was still unrecognizable from the swelling. We told him he could help Alex get better by drawing pictures to cheer him up. He made enough pictures to cover several bed spaces. Marty stayed with us for the remainder of the hospitalization. He, too, talked to his unresponsive brother. He borrowed a line from a scene in his favorite movie, *Bambi*, when Bambi was wounded. "Get up," he would say to Alex. "You've got to get up." We bought him a doctor's kit. He raced around the hospital, always wearing his stethoscope and toting his doctor's bag. The staff started calling him "Dr. Marty Party."

Two and a half weeks after being admitted to the hospital, Alex was weaned off of the respirator and was finally breathing on his own. Naively, we had expected him to sit up and talk. It was our wedding anniversary and not at all the way I had expected it to be. The medical team had warned us that his convalescence would be slow, but his recovery was a lot slower than we had expected. He was semiconscious some of the time, but he couldn't talk, he couldn't lift his head, he couldn't focus his gaze on us, and we weren't even sure he could see. Sitting at his bedside and being positive became increasingly difficult.

As they weaned him off of sedation, he went through intense periods of drug withdrawal. His faint, throaty groans and incessant thrashing made him seem more like a colicky infant than my four-year-old son. Sometimes it helped to hold him in my lap, but it was a major production to move him and all of his medical equipment. He still had chest tubes draining out of each side of his lungs. There were catheters in each side of his neck and in his chest. He also had a nose tube, a urine catheter, and half a dozen tangled electrode leads. When his physicians admitted that they were concerned about how slowly he was coming out of the coma, we became very depressed. We had to remind ourselves constantly to think only a day at a time.

Four weeks after his initial hospitalization, it was decided that Alex's psychological and neurological recovery would be better outside the intensive care unit. By this time, most of his tubes had been removed, and his sedation had been shifted to methadone. Alex had become a legend in the hospital, and it was with considerable apprehension that the head nurse admitted him on the medical floor. I didn't help matters much by accidentally hitting the CODE button rather than the NURSE CALL button within the first ten minutes of our arrival. The poor woman, whose face was drained of color, came barreling into the room, along with every other nearby nurse. The move did a lot for our spirits. After the noise, intensity, and pathos of the critical care unit, the medical floor felt like a rest home despite the cystic fibrosis kids Rollerblading down the hall.

Several days later, Alex spoke for the first time. When we asked him if he was going to get a puppy, he answered with a weak but definitive "yes." Now awake and conscious most of the day, the only things that seemed to console him were listening to Beethoven's *Archduke Trio* and listening to stories read over and over. Most of his organs slowly returned to normal with the exception of his kidneys. Every other day, we had to wheel him to the kidney dialysis unit for treatment. It was usually a tedious, three-hour process that made him freezing cold and left us all irritable. When his kidneys showed signs of restarting several weeks later, it was a tremendous relief, for it meant he no longer had to stay in Boston.

Day by day he was weaned off methadone and other sedatives. His agitation lessened and his vision seemed to improve. However, he still lacked the strength to hold up his head or to attempt to eat. We kept reminding him of the puppy. Soon you will be well and going home, we told him. We tried not to think about the possibility that he might never fully recover. It had been six long weeks. His speech was limited to "yes," and he had the muscular control of a quadraplegic. When he finally spoke his second word, it was "Vermont," and we knew that he now had a concept of going home. Psychologically, that was a major turning point for him.

By the time he left Boston, he was clearly saying "Go home." That was what we all wanted. Plans were made to move him back to the regional medical center for approximately two more weeks of convalescence. It would be closer to home for us, and he would be seen by physicians who would continue to monitor his long-term recovery. The day we left, he was loaded into an ambulance to make the three-hour trip back to Dartmouth-Hitchcock Medical Center. This time there was no urgency, no blinking lights, and no haunting sirens. There was just one very weak but happy boy. I propped him up on the stretcher so he could see out the back window, and I sat beside him. As we drove north on the interstate, I pointed out the tall buildings receding in the distance. Tears streamed down my cheeks. For nearly two months I had suppressed the thought, the fear, that this day might never happen.

Back at Dartmouth-Hitchcock he received physical therapy services and began eating again. As the effects of long-term sedation and bed rest wore off, he grew stronger and stronger. One week later, wobbly but remarkably determined, he walked out of the hospital holding our hands. He didn't forget the puppy. A dog was the first thing he asked for when he got home.

When we returned to Vermont, I began calling around to find a litter of golden retriever puppies. Luckily, I located a litter of twelve puppies in Westminster West, only about a half-hour drive from our home. The breeder told me that she had three puppies left that would be ready to go in a week and suggested I come over to see them. Tom was in New York on business at the time, so I called him and told him I wasn't going to buy a puppy; I was only going to take the boys over to look at them. Right.

As I got out of the car at the breeder's house, I was immediately greeted by a tangle of a dozen tan, playful puppies, lapping at my feet like waves of fur. The boys were in the backseat of the car, clamoring to get out, but they didn't quite know whether to dive into all the commotion or run away in fear. The breeder suggested that I sit Alex and Marty on a nearby picnic table, where we could try out the three remaining puppies, one by one. She scooped up the first puppy and handed him to me. He nipped at my fingers and squirmed so much I could barely hold him. "A bit antsy," I thought. Then she passed me the second puppy, who just froze and shook with fear when I sat him on the table. "If he thinks he's scared now," I thought, "wait until he's been chased endlessly by the likes of Alex and Marty."

The third puppy she captured was the runt of the litter, and he was a little darker than the rest, with a coat the color of fallen leaves. He seemed so peaceful when I held him that I reached over and placed the puppy on Alex's lap. The connection was instant. Alex's whole body relaxed, and from under his shaggy, overgrown bangs, his deep brown eyes were round with wonderment. It was the old Alex I knew before the illness. He cuddled the puppy, ran his fingers through his silklike fur, and marveled at his tiny floppy ears and wet spot of a nose. The puppy didn't scratch or squirm or nip, he just curled up in a ball and went to sleep. In a faint but joyous voice, Alex announced, "Him curly!" And so it was that "Curly," a wonderfully serene dog, came into our lives. To this day, Curly has been as much a part of Alex's recovery as any physician.

Beginning the Healing Journey

You are probably reading this book because you have a seriously ill or injured child or have been touched in some way by the struggle of a child to heal. You may be a family member, a close friend, a medical professional, or a hospital worker, but it doesn't really matter. All of us have the same goals in mind when it comes to nursing a child back to health—we want to do what is best for the child and the family, we want to heal in a way that causes the least hurt, and we want to make the right decisions so that we may be at peace with ourselves.

When Alex contracted the *E. coli* bug, Tom and I didn't realize we were embarking on a journey to the far reaches of the mind, the spirit, and medical technology. There were few signposts along the way. Instead, we were guided by our love for our son, our intuition, and our belief that something positive could always be found in a horrible situation. We discovered a whole constellation of knowledge out there—things that were not written down, things that were thought but never said, and feelings that transcended the best that medicine had to offer. We met a lot of other travelers along the way—parents who had been through far more arduous journeys, parents whose journeys paralleled ours, and parents who had abandoned any hope of recovery. We helped them to heal as they helped us. *More than anything, we learned that parents are every bit as important to healing children as medical professionals are.*

This book is about our personal healing journey with Alex, which is still far from over. His courage to survive and the incredible love generated by him were an inspiration to all of us who shared in Alex's miraculous recovery. Throughout the many days and nights Tom and I spent with Alex, waiting, hoping, and praying, I often thought about sharing what we had learned with other parents. As you begin your journey, I hope our story—our periods of joy and devastation, our hopes and our miracles, and our moments of insight and indecision—will help you guide your child through the healing process.

We always found that we had more questions than answers. Big questions, like:

- What should I look for in a physician?
- What can I as a parent do and not do?
- How do I develop trust in the medical team treating my child?
- Does my presence make a difference?
- How important is the attitude of the medical staff?
- Does my child understand what is going on?
- Why is faith such an important part of the healing process?
- How do I broach difficult ethical questions?

Throughout this book, I attempt to answer these questions, not as a professional, but as a parent.

We also had questions I couldn't even begin to attempt to answer, questions we will always ask, like:

- Why did this happen to me and my family?
- Why did my child survive while others who receive the same loving care do not?
- Is my child's soul inseparable in some ways from mine?
- Why has our suffering made us tender rather than bitter?

The questions didn't end when Alex survived. But, it was then that we made the astounding discovery that healing and recovery were not the same. Recovery, as difficult as it was for Alex, wasn't an endpoint; it was only a milestone in the healing journey. Alex is alive, and he's walking, talking, and just being Alex again, but the healing process—coping, adapting, and coming to terms with ourselves and others—has taken far longer. You, too, will discover the many issues ahead of you concerning siblings, families, friends, schools, playmates, and the tough decisions you must make about your family, your finances, and your careers. If this book helps make that process just a little easier, I have succeeded in what I set out to do.

Using This Book

You can either read this book from cover to cover or skip around from topic to topic. If you have recently had to face the problem of caring for an ill or injured child, you might want to skip right to chapter 3, "Taking Control," before reading on. It is meant to give you an overview of what you, the parent, *can* do. Has your child made it through an acute illness only to find that he or she has a lifelong chronic illness? You are not alone, as you will discover in chapter 11, "The Hidden Lives of Children with Medical Conditions." Maybe you are not the parent but a close friend or family member. What can you do to help? Chapter 14, "For Extended Family Members and Friends," will give you an insight into what the family might be thinking and feeling and how you can become a more effective means of support.

Come join us on our journey. Let us help you in the healing process.

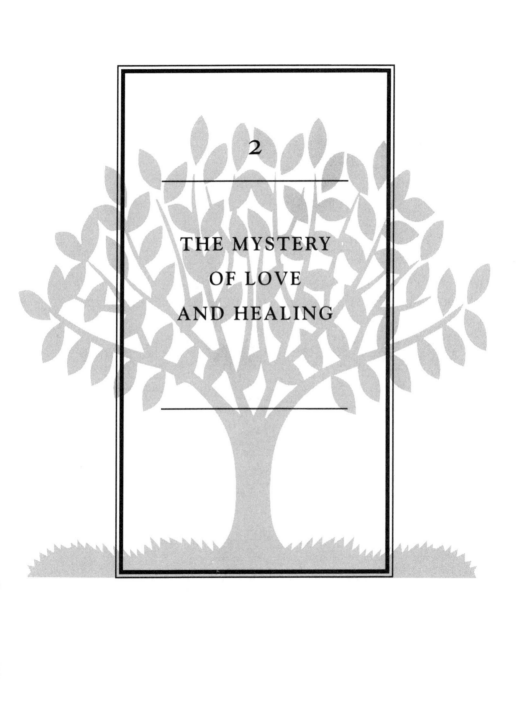

2

THE MYSTERY
OF LOVE
AND HEALING

For my twenty-first birthday, Tom bought me a cornstalk plant. We were seniors in college and we had been out shopping in downtown New Orleans. Walking down the sidewalk, we came upon a Woolworth's store with lush greenhouse plants practically spilling into the street. Impulsively, he picked out the most regal plant of all and bought it for me. It was flawless—no blemishes, no dead leaves, and perfectly shaped. I proudly carried it down the street and held it awkwardly in my lap on the city bus as we rode back to campus. It sat gloriously by the French doors of my dorm room throughout my senior year, and it was sitting there eavesdropping when Tom and I decided to get married. It was one of the few possessions that *had* to fit in our VW Squareback when we left New Orleans and began the long trek northward to Philadelphia for graduate school.

That plant has been a part of us for over twenty-two years now. It has weathered ten moves, covering thousands of miles. It's been moved on a dolly, crammed in the back of U-Haul trucks among bicycles, and toted awkwardly down the street like a Christmas tree. But that plant has grown as we have grown. When we moved to a stately, oversize brownstone in Brooklyn, our cornstalk plant grew oversize, too. Soon it was pressing impatiently against the twelve-foot ceilings. "What are we going to do with that thing?" was a frequent topic of discussion, but we never seemed to find an answer. When I finally became pregnant with our first child, Alex, we hit upon a solution. In honor of his birth we would chop it down, root the top in water, and let it grow back.

The night I had Alex was filled with so many mixed emotions. He was delivered by C-section at 6:00 P.M. and all went well, but within minutes after his birth he began to shake and tremble and my blood pressure shot up. The delivery room attendant called for an emergency-transport incubator, and Alex was whisked out of the room. At one moment I was holding my baby for the first time, wondrously studying his face and marveling at his tiny fingernails. The next moment he was gone.

No one was quite sure what was wrong, but since he was showing some classic signs of cocaine addiction, I was quizzed unmercifully about whether I had taken any "medications" during my pregnancy. I felt like answering, "How could you be asking a new mother who spent five years trying to get pregnant these ridiculous questions?" But I was so weak, exhausted, and emotionally spent that I humored them by being civil. "No, none, nothing," I repeated almost mechanically. What I really wanted to say was, "Listen, I just gave birth to a child with problems. Don't you care how I feel? Couldn't I have a little, just a little, bit of sympathy, *please?*" My blood pressure soared again. I felt drained, lying helplessly on a hospital bed with a huge black cloud of the unknown draped over me like a shroud. Not only was my baby not perfect, but he was also off in the neonatal ICU, all alone, encased in a plastic box. The "what-to-expect" books for new mothers hadn't prepared me for this.

Tom didn't know what else to do but to sit by me, hold my hand, and try to reassure me that things would be okay in the morning. His voice said one thing, but his cold, clammy hands told me another—he was terrified, too. By 11:00 P.M., I was still in the recovery room and they had finally got my blood pressure under control. Alex would be monitored overnight in the neonatal ICU, so I told Tom to go home and get some rest. He leaned over and kissed and hugged me. As he walked out of the room, I called out after him, "Make sure you chop down the cornstalk plant before you go to bed tonight."

And so it was that Alex came into the world. He spent his first week in the neonatal ICU on display like a pheasant under glass. I spent it as a helpless mother, confined to bed for many days. Tom stayed by Alex's side every moment he could. He couldn't hold Alex, but he could stick his arm in the opening of the incubator. Alex quickly took to holding on to Tom's pinky finger as if he would never let go. If drugs were not the problem, the physicians reasoned, it must be a metabolic problem, so Alex was poked, prodded, observed, and subjected to all kinds of invasive tests. At the end of the week, the neonatologists proclaimed his tremulousness a "variant of normal" and sent us home. After a rocky beginning, Alex calmed down and began to thrive. So did the cornstalk plant. It took a long time to sprout roots, but soon it started to grow and flourish once again.

Four years later, the same cornstalk plant was sitting in our bedroom window when the EMS people charged into the room at 5:00 in the morning and carried Alex's nearly lifeless body to the ambulance. Two weeks later I went back into our bedroom again. The bedcoverings were in disarray, leftover glasses of dried-up Pedialyte were perched on the night table, and medical debris from the EMS technicians littered the floor. Over in the corner, the cornstalk plant was drooping seriously, and the leaves of its midsection were bright yellow and dying. The room might as well have had the stench of the plague. I hastily cleaned up the room, washed my hands twice with antibacterial soap and scalding water, and gave the cornstalk plant a long drink of water.

Just as Alex survived, so did the cornstalk plant. Alex will always wear the battle scars of his illness on his body. The long scar running down his belly like a zipper will fade some, but the illness will always linger in his mind. I wonder whether he will ever be able to say the words "death" and "dead" again. He has totally eliminated them from his vocabulary and never fails to substitute the word "happy" for the word "dead."

I'll never get over his illness either, but my scars are of a different sort. I'll probably always be more protective than other mothers—panicking at the first sign of diarrhea, less willing to let my children out of my sight, and forever trying to control the quality of their environment. Recently when Alex lost his first baby tooth (and apparently swallowed it), I was sure he had fallen on his face when I wasn't watching.

I'll never stop worrying whether something catastrophic will happen to my children again. The other night at bedtime, our younger son, Marty, said to Tom, "Daddy, I don't want to die." It was an innocent enough statement for a child who has been through what he has, but it left Tom wondering whether Marty knew something we didn't. It wasn't very rational, but we stayed up late analyzing what Marty had said, trying to reassure each other that it was just an innocent expression of fear. Our conversation led to the one we have often—will we ever get over the feeling of vulnerability, or has Alex's illness changed our perspective on life forever?

And, I'll never stop searching for a reason why Alex's illness happened to us in the first place—was it destined to be, or were we simply victims of random bad luck? Sometimes when I'm running alone at dusk on the dirt roads near our home, the questioning in my mind will begin. It takes over so completely that I find I have effortlessly traversed steep hills with my legs pumping away at a near gallop. I wish I knew the answer.

Yellow leaves never turn green again; they die. The cornstalk plant, which is nearly five feet tall now, has a leafless girdle around its midsection, but its top is emerald green and bouncy once again. In a way, Alex and the cornstalk plant match. I simply cannot look at that plant without thinking about Alex. Sometimes I look at it, searching for hidden signs of what the future will bring for him. Sometimes I look at it and get angry that someone I love so much had to suffer so. And sometimes I look at it and I am filled with love—with joy that my son, for whatever reason, was chosen to live.

The Circle of Love

There is no denying that an illness like Alex's is devastating, but a tremendous outpouring of love came from it. It was as if one giant circle of wonderful people joined hands—many of them strangers—from Vermont to New Hampshire to Boston and back. Volunteers, orderlies, physicians, nurses, and ambulance drivers reached out to one another with a single purpose—to save Alex's life. Why? Not because it was their job. Not because they felt sorry for him or us. I think it was because they looked down at our son hanging on by a thread as if it were their own child. They felt deeply the love that we as parents have for him and were inspired to give him everything they had. Some of these people have become part of Alex's extended family. He has grandmothers, a grandfather, aunts, uncles, cousins, and a few people who have become just as important as family to him because they cared, and continue to care, in a big way whether he lived or died.

Who would have thought that an ambulance driver would reach

out to me and tell me how much my son's life meant to him because he saw himself as a sickly child in Alex? Who would have imagined that an ICU night nurse would tenderly wash, coif, and blow-dry Alex's hair when it wasn't clear that he would live until the morning? Or that the sixty-plus employees of Faith Mountain, the company owned by my brother and his wife, would take it upon themselves to start each day during Alex's illness with a silent moment of prayer?

We expect a lot from our pediatrician, but we never dreamed she would drive three hours to Boston on her day off to let us cry on her shoulders. The next day, our minister did the same. Who would have thought that one of Alex's nurses would bring in her son's toys to entertain him and send him presents on Christmases to come? Or that Alex's former nanny would drop everything in her life and drive halfway across the United States to help out with his recovery? On Sunday mornings, you could practically hear the prayers resonating in the air for Alex. In churches, from Texas to South Carolina to Vermont, Catholics, Baptists, Methodists, and Congregationalists all said the same prayers—for Alex, a little boy they barely knew who had so much to live for and so little chance of living.

"I have many prayer warriors here in Mt. Pleasant and Charleston praying for Alex. We will expect a miracle!" wrote a woman I didn't even know. She had heard about Alex while heaping plates full of food alongside my mother as a volunteer for the local Meals-on-Wheels program. Also a survivor of a life-threatening illness, she took it upon herself to organize a prayer group for a child she'd never met, and then spent the time writing to comfort me.

We were overwhelmed by the expressions of love for our child. It was as if the force of love and caring generated by all those people lifted him up above the pain and the misery and breathed life into him. I'll always wonder whether he pulled through because he had a reason to, because he felt the intense love radiating from that circle of people around him. As a parent, I'll also always question what force had pulled them all toward us. Were Tom and I two loving individuals who had made a difference, were we the force that brought all the people helping him together? In retrospect, I *think* we were. Had I known at the time, I'm not sure I wouldn't have collapsed under the weight of the responsibility. I didn't have much time to think—I just did what I felt in my gut was right. I asked people to push themselves and medical science to the limit, and they did.

Not all that long ago, a similar thing happened again on a much smaller scale. It was around dinnertime on Saturday evening when the phone rang. I was closest, so I answered it. On the other end was a woman so clearly panicked she could barely talk. It turned out that it was one of the housemates of our baby-sitter.

"Our roommate is having a real big seizure—we don't know what to do. We thought you'd know because of Alex. Oh, help us," she wailed.

Without even thinking, I told them to get him on his side and to extend his neck so his airway was open. She screamed my directions into the living room, where our baby-sitter and her husband were trying to help. I then told her to call EMS. She said she had; they were on their way. She hastily thanked me and hung up.

About an hour and a half later, just as we were about to put the kids to bed, the phone rang a second time. It was our baby-sitter's husband calling from the hospital to thank me again and to tell me their roommate was okay. I mumbled something along the lines of, "I really didn't do anything—I felt bad I couldn't be of any more help." On the contrary, he said, my directions were essential because their roommate was on his back, his skin was bluish-black, and he couldn't breathe when they called me. My directions helped them to get him breathing again, he said. By the time the ambulance arrived, their roommate was dazed and confused, but the seizure had stopped. I briefly relayed what he had told me to Tom. Then I took Marty upstairs to bed. I lay down on the bed in the dark next to Marty to kiss him good night. I paused there for a minute, and then it hit me. "My God," I thought. "I think I just helped save that guy's life." I wondered whether I would have given the same calm directions if I had known the guy was bluish-black and not breathing. I hope so, but I'll never know. Just as with Alex, I did what felt right at the time.

In emergency situations, people do amazing things. It is a tremendous thought to know that there are so many extraordinary people in the world. I'd like to think that the circle of love created by Alex's illness is still there. When I look out over Cooper Hill from our house and see all the way to Mount Monadnock in New Hampshire, I imagine the circle of love hovering along the ridges and above the mountaintops—a circle of love that will be there for the next child and all of the other children to come. As I sit here writing this book, I feel compelled to complete that circle of love by reaching out to other parents in similar circumstances.

"You Never Gave Up. . . . And Neither Did We"

The Christmas after Alex's illness, we got a card from a family we had met at the hospital in Boston. Things were looking up for them. Their six-year-old boy, Zach, had undergone neurosurgery for a seizure disorder at the time Alex was in Boston. For the first time in nearly two years, his seizures looked like they were under control. I got the chills when I read the letter, for we had been through terrible times together. We had cried countless hours together, we had recounted the horrors of the ICU every day for nearly a month, and now it seemed, finally, that both of our families were on the mend. Two days later I got a second letter.

"Guess where we are spending Christmas this year?" Laura wrote. "Not at home as I bragged in my last letter, but back in children's ICU in the *same* bed space as the summer. . . . I was in the parents' room yesterday and really wished you were there to talk to! Of course, I would never wish *that* on you!"

All the joy I had felt came crashing to the floor. I kept rereading the letter through blurry eyes, hoping it would say something different, but it didn't. I almost felt guilty that Alex was recovering and her child wasn't. We decided several days after Christmas to drive to Boston and surprise Zach and his family with a visit. It was Alex's first trip back to Boston since his illness. He was overly excited about going to the "big city" and getting to ride on a subway train. He chattered on and on in the backseat, telling us every minute detail he could recall about trains, all the way to Boston. Four months after his illness, he was now much stronger and had gained back the 30 percent of his body weight he had lost.

We weren't sure what to expect as we walked up the sidewalk to the front entrance. Would Alex remember anything? Would he be frightened? It sure brought back memories for me—I was shivering despite being dressed in heavy winter clothes. He approached the automatic doors of the hospital like a child going to the zoo for the first time. We remarked to each other that he either didn't remember the hospital or had suppressed his memories. Then it dawned on us that he had never seen the front door of the hospital—he had arrived in critical condition by ambulance and had left in stable condition, but still by ambulance. The ambulance dock might have been more familiar to him.

By the time we got to the medical ICU, Alex still hadn't figured out where we were. To him, we were on an adventure in a strange place, more like a museum than a medical facility. He and Marty were bouncing around, zooming from one side of the corridor to another. Walking into the waiting area of medical ICU, we accidentally ran into the attending physician who had managed Alex's case. He stopped and froze in amazement, for the last time he saw him, Alex wasn't able to talk or even lift his head. "That can't be . . . is . . . is that Alex?" he asked from a distance.

Up until this point, Alex didn't seem to recognize his surroundings, but when he heard the physician's voice, his bubbly demeanor disappeared. Suddenly, it all seemed to come back to him. He backed up against my legs, his body rigid with fear. The physician lowered himself to Alex's level with arms outstretched and called his name. I held Alex's hand and led him stiff-legged over to greet the physician. When he gave Alex a giant hug, Alex melted in his arms and began chatting excitedly—Alex said he felt fine and he was all well now. The physician's eyes were misty as he looked unbelievingly at us and said, "You never gave up." Then he paused and added, "And neither did we." I nearly fell over as those words echoed in my mind.

"What if we hadn't fought so hard for our son's life?" I thought. "Would they have taken their cue from us and given up, too?" We talked for a few minutes and went on to visit Zach, who, thankfully, had been moved out of the ICU the day before. For the rest of our visit, though, the attending physician's statement haunted me and was always there in the back of my mind.

Whenever I wonder whether we were the force that brought Alex's medical team together, I think about what that physician said, *"You never gave up. . . . And neither did we."* I can only conclude that we must have made a huge difference in whether he lived or died. How precisely, we'll never really know. It's not something for which you can devise a formula, but it is very much what this book is about.

The Warm Glow of Tenderness

The January following his initial hospitalization with the *E. coli* bacteria, Alex went back to Dartmouth for the surgical reversal of his colostomy. He ended up in the hospital for the entire month. It was only by pushing things that we were able to go home on January 30, Marty's third birthday. We desperately wanted to have something normal in our lives—for our sake, but mostly for Marty's. One day during that stay, I was feeling down and decided to go for a walk to jump-start my mind. As I was walking by the entrance to the ICU, our social worker popped out of her office next door and asked me if I would do her a favor. There was a young couple, she told me, whose one-month-old infant was being transferred to Boston that evening from the pediatric ICU. Would I be willing to tell them about getting around Children's Hospital and finding temporary housing? She introduced me to a couple sitting outside the ICU. Suddenly I felt I was standing in front of a mirror looking at myself six months before. When I made eye contact with the mother, I think we both acknowledged that we knew a transfer to Children's was a last-ditch effort to save their child, just as it had been for us. But we didn't talk about that.

I tried the best I could to tell them everything I wished I had known when we were transferred to Boston. Like us, they lived in the country. They were nervous about going to a city hospital hours away from home, about how to afford a place to stay, and most of all about the quality of care their child would receive. We talked for a long time while they were waiting for the pediatric-transport ambulance. They listened intently to everything I said, but more than anything, they clung to the fact that my child had survived—that he came back on his feet, not in a pine box. Our greatest fear at the time had been whether Alex would make it to Boston alive. Theirs was the same. Seeing and talking to me gave them hope. That couple never knew it, but the conversation did a lot for me, too. It made me think how far Alex had come, *and it gave me hope for the future.*

Despite all that we have gone through and all that we have ahead of us, I am not bitter. Neither are nearly all of the other parents of seriously ill or injured children I've ever met. They have a compassion about them that is instantly recognized by other parents who have been there.

Not all that long ago, I had the occasion to be out in the woods with a real estate agent for a "perc" test—the process by which land is assessed for its ability to support a septic system. A backhoe is driven as far into the woods as necessary, and a soil engineer directs the operator to dig a number of six-foot-deep test pits. It was a freezing cold late-November morning. There I was, standing in the middle of a spectacular stand of white birch trees, watching the backhoe's shovel dig grave-sized holes in the forest floor. I'm not sure how we got talking, but I found myself telling the real estate agent, Paul, about how stressful Alex's medical problems have been.

"I know," he said. "I've been there." He really didn't have to say more, for I could see it in his eyes.

Paul told me the story of how his son was diagnosed with a rare form of muscular dystrophy when he was eighteen months old and was not expected to live past the age of five. When his son could no longer walk, he scooted around on a tricycle. It wasn't until his son went to school and had to use a wheelchair that he admitted he couldn't do all the things other kids could. As a father, Paul devoted his entire life to his child. His son died at age seventeen in Texas, just after competing in the Special Olympics and winning a number of gold medals. It was an incredibly beautiful story that left me fighting back tears.

Just as he finished the story, Tom arrived with the kids from school. To Alex, backhoes are right up there with ice cream, airplane rides, and cuddly bunnies. He scrambled through the woods to see the backhoe at work. Paul was instantly drawn to him. He took Alex by the hand closer to the backhoe, kneeled down beside him, and put his arm around him. Paul's curly white hair was backlit by the sun, bathing the two of them in a glow. Soon they were intensely discussing construction equipment, road building, and the like, and Alex was in ecstasy. It was one of the tenderest displays of affection I had ever seen.

Why does suffering tend to make us tender rather than bitter? I'm not sure anyone knows for sure. Recently, I watched portions of Children's Hospital's annual telethon on television. Zach, the little boy we visited in Boston, was being profiled for his courage to heal despite the ultimate removal of the entire right hemisphere of his brain. Toward the end of the telethon, the emcee focused the camera on the telephone banks and volunteers. Four women, all mothers of children with cancer, were sitting together. They had met while their children were hospitalized, and here they were again, selflessly volunteering together to help raise money for other children. They weren't at home, guarding their time with their families, they were giving and sharing with others. Why? For me, helping other parents is very much a part of my own healing process. I often see myself in them, and in helping them to cope, I work on my old wounds, the wounds I'm not sure will ever completely heal. In volunteering, these mothers were helping to heal themselves.

RECOVERY AND HEALING ARE NOT THE SAME

For over a year after Alex's illness, we were afraid to go anywhere. In January following his illness, he underwent surgery to reverse his colostomy, and it was extraordinarily hard on him. Following the surgery, he had several life-threatening, prolonged seizures in the hospital, in which he lost consciousness, his body became rigid, and he lost the ability to breathe on his own.

The brain is a complex organ, whose smooth functioning is dependent on electrical signals that pass from one brain cell to another. In the case of a tonic-clonic or grand mal seizure like Alex's, an abnormal electrical discharge in one area of the brain sets off a chain reaction that appears much like an overloaded circuit. Tonic-clonic seizures like Alex's are not uncommon, but his differ from most others in that they are not self-limiting—they will continue indefinitely. Without immediate medical intervention, his seizures will certainly lead to oxygen deprivation and death.

These weren't the first seizures Alex had ever had. He had two others when he was younger, but had been seizure-free for nearly two years before the *E. coli* infection. When the bacterial infection caused inflammation of his brain, we expected seizures to be a problem, but they weren't for a long time. We even naively thought he might have outgrown them, as do many preschool-aged children.

Now, for some reason, nearly a year after the bacterial infection, the seizures were back in full force. Although he was on maximum dosages of antiseizure medications, he started having unexplained seizures. Every time he had one, he lost consciousness, had breathing difficulties, and required medical intervention to bring the seizure under control. It was a problem that we lived so far out in the country. Our idyllic lifestyle on top of a mountain in the middle of ski country seemed like such a dream when we left the intensity of New York City. Now it was our worst nightmare. How could we manage Alex's condition so far away from sophisticated medical facilities?

We have a wonderful neurologist who worked with us and our pediatrician to develop a plan to have emergency medication and an oxygen tank available in our home. We were instructed to administer a large dosage of Ativan rectally to stop the seizure and then to assist Alex in breathing, if necessary, giving him oxygen until help arrived. Tom and I mentally rehearsed the drill over and over. We diligently wrote down step-by-step directions and emergency phone numbers on a card to be carried with the medication at all times. We called the local rescue squad and informed them of our son's condition. We drew a map and wrote very specific directions to our house so that all of their volunteers would know exactly how to get to our home. We followed all of this up in writing so there would be no possibility of miscommunication. The only thing we couldn't control was the weather. I couldn't sleep on nights when we had freezing rain or snowy conditions. I'd toss and turn all night and be grumpy in the morning, but I was always relieved that we had made it through yet another night and another storm.

As much as Tom and I had rehearsed the drill, we felt totally unprepared when the first seizure at home struck. Little things we hadn't thought of cropped up. We had a devil of a time getting the Ativan out of the tiny little pressurized vials (later we learned that you have to inject as much air into the vial as the amount of liquid you are drawing out). We didn't quite attach the syringe to the rectal tube correctly, so precious drops of Ativan dribbled on the floor and were wasted. And, we hadn't practiced the drill with Alex's younger brother bouncing around excited to "play doctor," asking questions, and demanding our attention (we learned to handle him by giving him an important job—to watch for the ambulance). Despite our feelings of ineptitude, Alex's seizure stopped after about twenty minutes, and the ambulance got him to the hospital smoothly for emergency follow-up care. That night we had the biggest blizzard of the year, and thirty inches of snow piled up everywhere. We barely scraped by.

Mysterious Tree Carvings and Other Thoughts

So, it was no wonder that we were afraid to travel. But after a summer of chicken pox and more hospitalizations, things seemed to calm down for Alex. Finally, we thought the time was right to get away—we really needed it for our own sanity. We arranged to stay with my mother at her home on the beach near Charleston, South Carolina. But before we traveled, I called the airline to see if we could bring a small oxygen tank with us. As I suspected, we couldn't. They could arrange to have a tank onboard for a charge of $50, but the problem was that the entire airline had only ten tanks and there was a six-month wait to have one available. We decided to chance it on the flight and to have my mother rent an oxygen tank in South Carolina for the duration of our stay. I felt fairly certain that if Alex had a seizure on the plane and his condition was life-threatening, they could make their emergency oxygen available. Even so, we carried resuscitation equipment (an ambu bag) onboard so that we could breathe for him manually if we had to. We also had my mother locate a reputable pediatric neurologist in Charleston, who agreed to be available for the duration of our stay.

We made the trip uneventfully, and it turned out to be fine for all of us. Alex and Marty tore out to the beach and spent hours collecting shells and building sand castles. Over the two-week period, we were able to relax for the first time in nearly a year. As Alex chased sandpipers up and down the beach and waded in knee-deep water, he grew stronger and more like his old self. Also for the first time since Alex's illness, my mother and I were able to talk openly about all that had happened. Sensing how fragile Tom and I were, she had avoided talking about a lot of her feelings and perceptions during the course of Alex's illness. I had been reading a lot about the nonmedical aspects of healing—about the importance of unconditional love and the will to live—and was eager to talk about how it related to Alex's illness. I had just read a provocative and compelling new book about scientific evidence for the power of prayer. I asked my mother whether she thought prayer could make a difference.

"I believe it, Nancy," she said. "There is something else out there. I feel it. I felt it when Alex was getting sick. I knew there was something wrong the moment I stepped off the plane, when he said, 'Grandma, go home.' I've always felt such a connection to him."

And then she told me about her dream the night that Alex nearly died—how she had been taking him by the hand down a tunnel to the outstretched hands of a man dressed in all black. She had been afraid to tell me about it all this time for fear that it might upset me.

"It doesn't matter what you call it," she said, and then almost as an afterthought, added, "You know, the Bible says that God is love. I think God's will is delivered through human hands." She got up to find the exact citation for me. There it was in I John 4:7–8:

> Beloved, let us love one another; for love is of God, and he
> who loves is born of God and knows God. He who does not
> love does not know God; for God is love.

I thought about what she said for a while and then stored it away with all of the rest of the information I was absorbing on the non-medical aspects of healing.

At the end of the two weeks, we flew back to Vermont, rejuvenated by the break in our routine, but glad to be home. Within a week of our return, Alex's seizures started all over again. It was so disheartening. Our whole life had been turned upside down for a year, and it seemed like it was never going to end. We finally made the decision that we both knew we had been avoiding all along. We needed a life beyond being armchair doctors and nurses and loving parents. We needed to pull up our roots and move closer to a medical facility where help was minutes rather than an hour away. Only then could we eliminate some of the daily stress of worrying, worrying, and more worrying. During the autumn, we started looking for a place closer to Brattleboro.

We decided to invite my family to spend the next, and our last, Christmas in our present home with us. My mother, one brother, and my sister and her husband agreed to come. Marty, the artistic one among us, took it upon himself to festively decorate our house. For weeks before Christmas, he busied himself making ornaments and decorations out of red and green macaroni, feathers, and cardboard. He drew pictures of green Christmas trees and plastered them all over the kitchen cabinets. But the thing he really wanted was a wreath with a great big red bow. I promised him that before Grandma came, we would get some pine boughs and make one.

It was the afternoon on the evening that my mother was to arrive that Marty reminded me that I had never got around to collecting the pine boughs to make a wreath. Alex and Marty were terribly excited about having visitors, particularly ones bringing presents, and had been full of energy all day. They were tearing around the house in anticipation. All I wanted was to make it through the evening without stitches from some nasty fall, so I agreed to take Marty down to cut some pine boughs near the beaver ponds in the woods below our house. The ground was covered with about eight inches of snow, so we decided to walk along the back of our property line next to the stream. It would be the quickest way to get there. Just as we reached the northeast corner of our land, Marty stopped abruptly.

"Come on, Marty," I said. "It's going to be dark soon." Then I noticed he was staring at a big beech tree on the corner of our property.

"Mommy, why are there letters on that tree?" he asked. I looked up, and there carved in big letters on the tree was the inscription GOD IS LOVE. This was not someplace like a subway stop, where you might see grafitti, nor were we close to any lover's lane, where someone might carve their initials. This was in the middle of the woods, in the middle of nowhere, on our land, and I had never noticed it before.

"That's really weird," I said out loud.

"What's weird, Mommy? What does it say?" he asked.

" 'God is love,' " I answered.

"What does it mean, Mommy?" he asked.

"I don't know. I wish I did," I answered.

"Why is it there on the tree?" he asked.

"I don't know that either," I said. "Let's go get those pine branches before it gets dark."

How could I begin to explain to a three-year-old how strange I felt—what an uncanny coincidence it was to see that message on a tree within minutes of my mother's arrival. And why was it on *our* land anyway? How could I explain to him something that even I couldn't begin to understand? To this day, I haven't found an explanation.

3

TAKING CONTROL

As a parent, you think that you can protect your children from anything. You can make them feel better when they hurt. You can comfort them when they are scared. You can cheer them up when they are sad. But when your child becomes seriously ill or is fighting for his or her life, you feel helpless. In a hospital, your usual parenting tasks are assumed by others or else become irrelevant. Feelings of vulnerability are heightened by the fact that you may not be permitted to see your child if his or her condition is unstable. You wait, you worry, you pace back and forth, you hope, and you pray.

Fortunately, most parents won't have to endure an experience as traumatic as our son's. Yet, each year approximately 2.5 million children become seriously ill or suffer injuries that require hospitalization. Regardless of the severity of your child's condition, hospitalization places significant stress on you, your child, and your entire family.

Loss of Control

When you are no longer in control of your child's well-being, you feel totally helpless. No matter what you do, you can't reverse what has happened. You alone cannot make your child well. Your sense of helplessness may be expressed by a range of emotions—confusion, denial, anger, guilt, grief, depression, and fear, to name a few. There is an unreality to what is happening. You find yourself repeating over and over, "It's not fair. Why me? Why my child? How can this be happening?" It is not uncommon to be angry. You may be angry at yourself, your physician, your child, or even God. Desperately, you look for someone or something to blame.

For a number of years, psychologists have been studying a phenomenon called "learned helplessness." People have a tendency to give up when placed in an aversive situation over which they have no control. They become highly stressed and learn to passively accept the difficult situation. For the parents of the hospitalized child, this poses two problems: You tend to withdraw from your child's recovery process, and you intensify the stress of an already stressful situation.

Learned helplessness can be a formidable enemy of both you and your child. Your child is seriously ill or injured and needs medical science to recover. But your child also needs your presence, your involvement, and your love to heal. You can't sit back and leave your child's fate in the hands of medical science. You have to fight your emotions and regain control of the situation.

How will you get through the next day? The next week? When will it all end? You must begin by adapting your role as parent to the hospital setting.

NINE STEPS FOR REGAINING CONTROL

1. Make yourself a member of your child's medical team.
2. Question, question, question.
3. Request a daily plan.
4. Request a short-term plan if your child's condition is critical.
5. Be there for your child.
6. Shift your time frame away from the future—live day to day.
7. Seek out and accept the support of others.
8. Manage contacts with extended family.
9. Take care of yourself.

It is your child lying in bed, and you are his or her best advocate. Read through the following steps for regaining control. Find those actions that meet your needs and the level of involvement you can handle. Start participating in your child's healing and recovery process.

1. Make yourself a member of your child's medical team.

In the beginning, faces seem to appear at your child's bedside at random. Although you may feel like a sideshow act in some perverse circus, these are the various members of the team becoming acquainted with your child. This team involves many people, including an attending physician responsible for the pediatric unit, a primary physician, a nurse, a respiratory therapist (if your child is on a ventilator or is having breathing difficulties), and a hospital social worker. As the person who knows your child best, you also are a critical team member. The team also may include fellows, residents, medical students, physical therapists, nutritionists, and child life specialists, depending on the institution and the complexity of the illness.

Remember that you are your child's best advocate. As soon as your child is settled, someone will probably debrief you on the status of your child. At this point, make yourself a member of the team. In most cases, you don't need to be pushy or aggressive. You just need to let the team coordinator know that you feel you are an essential part of the recovery process. Emphasize that your interest in your child goes beyond "Will my child be okay?" The more you ask questions, the more visible you are, and the more you offer valid observations, the more you will be involved in the management of your child's case.

Early on, ask to meet with the team leader or coordinator. Try to give a thorough, objective history of your child's condition. Discuss your concerns. Make clear what you hope to get accomplished as your child recovers. If your child is in very critical condition, you probably will be asked how much you want done for your child. Talk directly and openly. At some time, you may even be asked whether you want to withdraw your child's life support systems. Take your time to answer such questions, and don't let anyone try to influence the decision you need to make for yourself.

Find out who is on the team and why. What medical specialties are represented? Why are they involved in the management of your child's case? Since you meet so many faces in the beginning, don't be intimidated about asking them to reintroduce themselves. Ask the same questions of different team members. You may be surprised how much you can learn from the different perspectives.

Seek out people who tell you the facts, not just what you want to hear. As unfortunate as it may be, your interest in being a part of the medical team may be met with hostility in some settings. Seek out the person on the team that you find the easiest and most helpful to talk to. Use this person as a point person to offer and receive unbiased information to and from the team. A trusted team member, be it a nurse, a resident, or a social worker, will be an essential connection to your child's care.

2. Question, question, question.

It is not at all unusual to feel utterly confused at first. The shock of your child's sudden illness or injury, combined with the bombardment of information from various specialists, can be overwhelming. You may find it very difficult to listen to all that is being said. You may not be able to suppress your emotions enough to listen. You may find that you focus on certain details, but can't remember the rest. These are all natural reactions. Once you get over your initial confusion, you will need to ask many questions. One essential thing to remember is that *you can never ask too many questions— your child's well-being is at stake.*

Understand the reality of the situation. Everyone wants to hear that their child will be okay, but first and foremost, you need to accept the severity of your child's condition. Wait until you are over the initial shock of your child's illness so that you can talk unemotionally. Ask for a candid assessment of your child's prognosis and course of recovery. Ask about outcomes of other patients with similar illnesses and injuries. You need to trust that your physician either will give you a candid assessment of your child's condition or will tell you honestly that he or she doesn't know.

Ask questions about the medical equipment sustaining your child. Ask your nurse a simple question like, "What are all these things being used for?" This will usually result in a layperson's description of each piece of equipment. Your child may be hooked up to a monitor for tracking his or her vital signs. *Have the nurse explain the normal ranges of these vital signs for your child. Don't hesitate to ask why these values might be out of the normal range.*

Ask questions about the medication your child is receiving. Your child may have at least one intravenous (IV) line attached to his or her hands, arms, or legs. Hydrating fluids, as well as drip medications, are delivered to the bloodstream through this IV. Is your child in pain? What pain medications are being used? How do they know when to administer more pain medication? If your child is on a ventilator for breathing support, your child will probably be receiving a paralysis medication to immobilize him or her. If your child is awake and aware, the inability to move can be terrifying. How do they tell when the medication is wearing off?

Ask about the implications of your child's illness or injury. Will there be temporary or permanent neurological damage? Will there be temporary or permanent damage to any internal organ or bone structure? Will your child have temporary or permanent physical disabilities? Is there a typical length of the recovery period? Bear in mind, though, that changing conditions may mean that these answers might change. Also understand that sometimes "I don't know" is the best answer that they can give you.

Ask for written material if you don't understand something or want to know more about your child's condition. Most hospitals have fairly simply written descriptions of illnesses and injuries they can give you. If you want to read in more detail, ask for recent medical or nursing journal articles on the topic. Many teaching hospitals have medical libraries on the premises, if you choose to research a topic on your own.

Try to make your questions as specific as possible. Open-ended questions such as, "How's she doing?" "Is she doing better?" or "Is she going to be okay?" usually result in general answers and may not give you a satisfactory reply. Once you understand more of the details of your child's condition, ask specific questions, such as, "Is

her blood pressure coming down?" or "Is her breathing still labored?" *Specific questions will yield answers that provide a far more
realistic snapshot of your child's condition.*

3. Request a daily plan.

Every morning doctors make rounds. During this process, a group of
doctors literally walks around the unit from bed to bed and dis-
cusses each case. Typically, one physician who has studied the last
twenty-four hours of data on your child will present the case. Often,
if you are at the bedside, they will seek your input, so it is very important to try to be with your child during morning rounds. After the
rounds, physicians meet with your nurse and discuss how they intend
to proceed with your child's treatment. At this point, they work out
the beginnings of a plan for the day. You have a right to be de-
briefed on the plan, but sometimes you must ask specifically what will
happen to your child that day. If you don't ask, you might find
yourself spending the day waiting for something to happen, wondering what they are going to do for your child. Not knowing what
will happen will only increase your sense of helplessness.

Ask about the tests to be done that day. What tests will be done on
your child? Why will these tests be done, and what do they expect
to learn from the results? When will the tests be done? Where will
the tests be done? Will the tests or sedation associated with the
tests have observable effects on your child? When will the test results be available and who will explain the results?

Ask about new or different medications. Will they try higher or
lower levels of medication or different medication schedules today?
Are any new medications going to be tried? Can you expect to see
any behavioral changes associated with shifts in medication?

Ask how they will manage your child's case today. Particularly if your child is in a pediatric ICU, things change daily, and even hourly. What new or different things will they try that day? For example, will they attempt to wean your child off the respirator? Will they try to lower oxygen concentrations? What is their logic for trying something new or different?

4. Request a short-term plan if your child's condition is critical.

Managing a serious illness or injury may involve considerable problem solving just to keep the patient going until a treatment or cure can be administered. As an ICU physician in a children's hospital directly stated, "Much of what we do is a futile attempt to stave off the inevitable." Working against the odds or in spite of the odds requires a thorough plan that can be executed quickly. You should be a part of the plan from the onset. If your child's condition is very critical, you need to be available to give written permission for any invasive procedure. If you are not nearby, make sure that you are always notified of any shifts in strategy. There may be many, depending on your child's condition.

Ask for an explanation of the strategy to be used for managing your child's case. What is going to happen over the next several days or week? What assessments need to be made? What treatments need to be administered? What diagnostic tests will be used and what will they tell you?

Outline the questions of concern to you, and make the team aware of the time frame in which you need answers. Initially, physicians focus their efforts on sustaining your child's life. As a result, they may let specific questions go unanswered for a period of time. However, you need to be insistent if you have serious concerns. For example, you might want an assessment of your child's level of cognitive functioning before proceeding any further. Recognize, though, that it is not always possible to balance your needs with those of medical science.

Ask when you will know whether your child is likely to recover. Don't be afraid to ask your team coordinator to commit to some time frame. Psychologically, this will give you a time period in which to sort out your thoughts and emotions. Many times, however, the physician cannot or will not give you a definite answer, but it doesn't hurt to ask.

Ask what changes might be expected in the short run. Do they expect to see immediate changes or gradual changes over a period of time? Will those changes be obvious? What might you look for as a parent?

5. Be there for your child.

One of the most important things you can do for your child is to be at his or her bedside. Even if your child is in a coma, anesthetized, or heavily sedated, talk to and touch your child. Recent studies have shown that auditory and tactile stimulation have a significant effect on recovery. Unconscious patients appear to be able to hear, even though they may not appear to respond behaviorally. Support for this argument comes from the fact that anesthesia does not necessarily affect the auditory pathways to the brain, including the auditory cortex, where the brain interprets the meaning of the words. Healing messages have the greatest effect when they are meaningful; hence *your presence and the positive messages you give are of utmost importance to your child.*

Be with your child as often as you can. Most pediatric units allow one parent to be with his or her child all the time. However, if your child is in the ICU setting, you may have to be fairly aggressive about being with your child. Typically, you are not allowed in an ICU when a "procedure" is in progress, or when a new patient is being admitted, nursing shifts are changing, or doctors are making their rounds. They may also ask you to leave if a nearby patient is in a crisis mode. In reality, these situations account for a great deal of time. You need to visit your child without obstructing the work of the professional staff. However, it doesn't hurt to remind the staff if you have been waiting for a significant length of time—sometimes they get distracted and forget about you.

Talk positively to your child. The sound of your voice is tremendous healing therapy for your child. Try to talk to your child in words that are meaningful and understandable to him or her. Different age children will have a different understanding of what is happening to them. Don't feel bad if you find it difficult to continue talking to an unresponsive child. That is natural. Read stories or poetry to your child. I read poems by Robert Frost to my unconscious four-year-old. He may not have understood them, but I'm certain he was soothed by the sound of my voice and the melodic lines of the poetry (and it made me feel better!). When you leave your child's bedside, let him or her know that you are leaving and will return soon. And, when you are not at the bedside, leave a tape recorder at the head of your child's bed, softly playing familiar tapes. Recent studies have demonstrated that music eases anxiety, stress, and pain in both children and adults, even in a coma.

Remind your child about what is happening each time you visit. Many seriously ill children are sedated with medication that has memory-blocking properties. The good news is that your child probably won't remember his or her hospital stay. The bad news is that every time you visit, you may have to remind your child where he or she is and what is happening. This will lower his or her anxiety and confusion level. Even though my child was unconscious, I could tell when he was awake, for a teardrop often formed at the corner of his eye when he heard me explain that he was very sick and lying in a hospital bed.

Touch, caress, and hold your child. Try to make physical contact with your child as much as possible. This may be fairly easy if your child has a room on the unit. But, if your child is in a pediatric ICU, you may be intimidated by the amount of medical equipment, tubes, etc. Ask the nurse if you are unsure of where to touch or caress your child. If your child is not on a respirator, most ICUs will allow you to hold your child in your lap if he or she is small enough. Make sure that you are in a comfortable chair with lots of pillows and in a comfortable position. It usually takes a great deal of effort to move a child with tubes, suctions, monitor leads, and the like attached. Be prepared to stay put until someone can assist you in placing your child back in the bed.

Bring familiar objects to your child's bedside. Make sure to bring a familiar, soothing object for your child, even if your child is in the ICU. It may be your child's favorite stuffed animal, a blanket, or a pillow. A child will find comfort in the touch, smell, and sound of familiar objects. Put up a current picture of your child in the bed space. Since the staff only see your child when he or she is ill, they respond very positively to a picture of the healthy child. This positive energy can only spill over into the overall healing of your child.

Talk positively about your child. Even if your child does not understand what is being said, avoid talking negatively about your child or your child's condition. Negative messages have been demonstrated to have an overall detrimental effect on the duration of recovery. Most physicians and nurses are careful not to talk explicitly in front of patients, but don't hesitate to remind someone. Spell if you must convey negative information—people around you will get the picture. To this day, it makes me clench my fists just to think of the surgical resident who announced in front of my *awake* four-year-old child, "God, I was sure he was going to die!" I'm sure she thought a four-year-old wouldn't understand. It happened so unexpectedly, I couldn't stop her. Be on guard, for this is an example of the unbelievable ignorance that even trained pediatric professionals can exhibit.

6. Shift your time frame away from the future—live day to day.

It is very natural to let your mind race ahead and worry about the future. What if my child doesn't recover? What if my child lives and is disabled for life? How will I ever cope? Worrying about the future causes even more anxiety than the reality of your child's illness or injury. You can optimize your child's chances of full recovery, but you can't control the future. When you start thinking about the future, you're placing yourself back in an uncontrollable situation.

Redefine the future according to severity of illness. Many parents have found that the best way to cope with their intense anxiety over the future is to shift their focus away from the big picture to what they can do today. Depending on the nature of your child's illness or injury, simply try to get through the next hour, the next day, or the next week. Stop yourself every time your mind drifts to pondering the future. As you achieve each milestone, set your sights a little more to the future. An ICU resident once told us about our critically ill child, "He and he alone will tell us which way he is going." We waited hour by hour and day by day for him to signal his direction. Only when it was apparent that he might recover did we begin to define the future beyond twenty-four hours.

Learn positive and negative indicators. Medical professionals look at the whole person. However, for most illnesses and injuries, physicians track one or more indicators of improvement and decline. Some indicators may be obvious, such as increased heart rate, but others such as calcium levels or blood gas levels may require additional testing. Although indicators cannot be tracked out of context, you will have a better sense of how your child is doing if you understand what the physicians are looking for. Ask someone on the medical team to explain the main indicators, both positive and negative, for your child's illness. Review the status of these indicators every morning before discussing the day's plan for your child. When my son was critically ill, his kidneys failed. Certain blood levels were checked daily to evaluate his kidney function, as was his urine output. The first sign that his kidneys were restarting, we were told, would be increased urine output. Every morning we asked about the levels and checked his catheter tube for urine. We cheered for him the morning a few drops of urine first appeared, for we knew the recovery process had begun.

Don't hesitate to call something unusual to the staff's attention. You see your child every day and know him or her better than anyone else. Nursing staff may change, physicians may rotate to different areas, but you are always the parent. You have a point of view that cannot be duplicated by any professional. If you think you see something unusual, *never* hesitate to call it to the staff's attention. *Nuances in behavior or subtle shifts in vital indicators may be apparent to you well before they are noticed by the medical team.*

7. Seek out and accept the support of others.

When you're still trying to deal with the reality of your hospitalized child, it is easy to ignore the various support services hospitals have to offer. Most hospitals provide professional support for parents in the form of chaplains, social workers, and trained volunteers. You will also receive offers of support from friends, relatives, coworkers, and most immediately, the parents of other children in the unit. Don't ignore these offers of support; they can help you tremendously in alleviating stress.

Utilize the hospital's support services. When your child is seriously ill or injured, you have more than enough stress to deal with. You shouldn't have to concern yourself with financial matters, housing problems (if you are away from home), and transportation. All hospitals have professional support to assist you with these types of issues. Soon after your child is admitted, a hospital social worker will visit you. Think about those areas in which you could use assistance. Don't be shy about asking for help if it will make your life a little easier. Some hospitals may also have child life specialists who can provide aid in dealing with your child and his or her siblings. Finally, don't overlook the hospital chaplains. In addition to offering you spiritual support and a sympathetic ear, they can provide a link to your home church or synagogue and its support network.

Screen offers of support to ensure they are adding rather than subtracting energy. Many people will ask how they can help you. Be careful not to stress yourself more by feeling that you have to talk with everyone who calls. Think of ways that people can help you at a distance. Support can be direct, like providing transportation, checking on your house, mowing your lawn, shoveling snow, or sitting with your child while you attend to critical business. Support can also be indirect, like offering prayers, giving blood, or conveying information on your child's status to others.

Accept support from and give support to other parents in similar situations. As soon as your child is settled in his or her bed, you will discover that you are not alone. Around you will be other parents with seriously ill or injured children. These parents, more than anyone else, understand how you are feeling. Particularly in a pediatric ICU, events such as the death of a child in a nearby bed space are very upsetting. The support of other parents can help you through these times. It can also be very therapeutic to talk to them about what is happening to your child. You'll be surprised how much information about the hospital, the staff, and coping with a child's illness that you can learn from comparing notes with other parents. Try to be a sympathetic listener as well. *As you help other parents cope, you will gather inner strength for yourself.*

8. *Manage contacts with extended family.*

It is only natural for close family members and friends to want to help you in a time of crisis. However, if your child is critically ill, the situation may be very tenuous during the early days of your child's illness. For some parents, having other people around can add even more stress. Figure out a level of support that is comfortable for you, and don't be shy about making your position known to your family and friends.

Keep calls and visits from concerned persons at a minimum. If your child is seriously ill or injured, calls and visits may add to an already stressful situation. As your child recovers, however, these calls and visits can hasten the recovery process. If your child is in an ICU, usually only two people are allowed to visit a child's bedside at the same time. This is to minimize stress on the critically ill child as well as other children in the unit. Most ICUs also limit visits to immediate family members. Ask non–family members to wait until your child is moved to a regular pediatric ward before planning a visit. It is also often difficult to receive phone calls in an ICU setting. Minimize incoming calls by assuring your family and friends that you will regularly update them on the status of your child.

Appoint a spokesperson(s) to convey critical information to family members and others. When your child is critically ill and his or her condition can change from hour to hour, family members and friends will want to stay in close touch. Making many calls each night and explaining your child's condition over and over can be both costly and wearing. Rather, appoint one or more family members as the spokesperson(s). Call that person as often as necessary, update him or her on the status of your child, and ask him or her to relay the information to the rest of the family.

Minimize your worries on the outside. Make sure that siblings, your house, pets, etc., are secure with family members or others you trust. With all the stress you are under, you shouldn't have to worry about additional matters such as these.

Don't be too proud to accept financial assistance from family or others. At first, it is difficult to assess the financial impact of your child's illness on your family. If you are offered financial assistance, do not reject the offers, for sometimes the ultimate cost of your child's illness can be enormous. Even though you may be insured, there may be dollar amount caps on the amount of your insurance coverage. In addition, there are many costs that are not covered by insurance. For example, you may find that your child requires additional medical equipment once he or she is released, which is not covered by your policy. If your child is hospitalized away from home, you may encounter transportation and parking costs, housing expenses, costs for meals, and expenses associated with babysitters for siblings. If your child's illness is lengthy, you may even find that you must take a leave of absence without pay from your job. All of these expenditures can add up and provide an additional level of stress that you don't need.

9. *Take care of yourself.*

Managing your child's hospitalization puts an incredible strain on you and your family. Your endurance is pushed to the limit, the emotional exhaustion is overwhelming, and you have to make critical decisions under stress. During this time more than ever, your child needs for you to be strong. "How do you keep going?" people ask. "I don't know," you answer. "I don't have a choice." It is important to maintain your stamina and your psychological health. *You do that by taking care of yourself.*

Take time off from your work to be with your child. Everyone's situation is different, but if you possibly can, take some time off work to be with your child. This is particularly important in the beginning, when your child's condition may be the most critical. Most employers will be understanding under the circumstances. The recently passed Parental Leave Act provides for three months of unpaid leave, with a guarantee of reemployment, for situations just like this. *You will never regret the time not spent at work, but you will always regret the time not spent with your child.*

Eat regularly and get sufficient sleep. It is not easy to eat high-quality food at normal times of the day in a hospital setting. As much as possible, try to eat a balanced diet and eat regularly. You need the energy, and you need the regular breaks from the ICU setting. As long as you stay in the hospital, someone can always reach you in an emergency. Having a child in the hospital is synonymous with sleep deprivation. Do the best you can to keep on a normal schedule. Go to bed at the same time every night, and rise in time to meet with the medical team as it makes its early morning rounds.

Find time for yourself. It is important to take some time for yourself so that you don't burn out. If your child is critically ill and you are anxious about leaving your child's bedside, ask if the ICU has a beeper for use by parents. Or, you can call in frequently to check on your child. Try to find some way to relax—read, exercise, listen to music, take an hour to go to a museum. Do whatever works best for you. During one winter hospitalization, our ICU physician suggested we take a few hours off and ski at the local ski mountain. It was a terrific suggestion, for it totally recharged us to be outdoors, away from the intensity of the ICU.

Keep communication with your spouse open. A hospitalized child puts undue stress on even the best relationship. Try your best to talk through your emotions. Try not to blame each other or yourself for your child's illness or injury, whatever the cause. If you need additional professional help in dealing with your feelings, ask to meet with the hospital social worker or consider therapy or counseling. Between you and your spouse, try as best you can to balance the burden of staying at the hospital and managing your life on the outside. Always keep in mind the two of you may have very different responses to the stress of the situation. Try to accept your spouse's response as nonjudgmentally as possible.

4

HEALING THROUGH
TEAMWORK

About six months after Alex was released from the hospital with the *E. coli* infection, I was driving the kids to preschool one day. It was the height of mud season, that time of year only Vermonters can appreciate, when the brown, gooey stuff is everywhere—spread like thick frosting on every road, tracked throughout your house, and even caked in your child's hair. The roads seemed firm enough that day, so I decided to go the back way on Upper Dover Road. Up ahead I saw a pickup truck coming toward me. We both instinctively moved to the right. Just as we were about to pass each other, it happened. *Thuwuup.* In an instant we were both stuck, really stuck. The whole right side of my car sank down into the mud up to the top of the wheels. Marty and Alex, who were strapped in their car seats, started to panic, for they were now pitched sideways.

I got out and dragged the two boys out on my side of the car, working against gravity. Together, the other driver and I assessed our predicament. We were stranded on a back road with no houses around and our vehicles had the road totally blocked. We rummaged around in the back of his truck, found a few short planks to shove under the back wheels, and managed to get his truck out of the mud. He then offered to go and borrow a bigger truck to tow us out. We passed the time by stomping and squishing about in the muddy gullies that ran down the road, singing as loud as we could. When the other driver returned, he towed us out, and we continued on our way to school, only about an hour late.

When we got home at the end of the day, I said, "Hey, guys, tell Daddy what happened on the way to school."

"We got really stuck, Daddy. We sunk the car," Marty said.

"Really?" said Tom. "How did you get out?"

Alex spontaneously answered, "Dr. Karen fixed it, Daddy. Dr. Karen got us out of the mud."

Some kids worship caped crusaders or futuristic wonder kids, but not Alex. Alex's hero is Dr. Karen, his pediatrician, and in his fantasy world, he attributes unearthly powers to her. It was Dr. Karen's skill in the emergency room and Dr. Karen's insight on that fateful morning that saved his life. The most amazing thing is, despite the fact he was only four years old at the time, he knows it. To him, Dr. Karen is superhuman. In his imagination, she can do anything—even willing our car from the jaws of Upper Dover Road. The story of our son's healing team begins with her.

She Promised Me She Would Be There

At 4:00 on the morning we called the ambulance, Karen was not on call. A new pediatrician, whom we barely knew, was covering emergency pediatric cases. For some reason I'll never know, I ran to the phone just as the ambulance pulled away with Tom and Alex inside, and made another call to the pediatrician on duty. I was crying and barely able to get the words out, but I begged as only a distraught mother could for her to call Karen. Karen had only recently become our pediatrician. One of the reasons we chose her was that she had trained in emergency pediatrics at a big city hospital. "She *promised* me she would be there if we ever had an emergency," I wailed. And she was, for the story of my son's healing team began not only with Karen, but also with us, the parents, for recognizing the severity of the situation and insisting that someone we knew and trusted be in charge.

You probably put a lot of thought into choosing a pediatrician. I know we did. Having faced some medical crises early in Alex's life, we knew we wanted a pediatrician who worked well under stress and who was willing to refer us to specialists when the answers were not obvious. We wanted someone we respected and the kids liked. We wanted someone who would treat our children as persons, not just two more stuffy noses and ear infections. *But most of all, we wanted a pediatrician who valued our intuition as much as his or hers.* Karen is that person. We think alike. We problem-solve together, and I think we are about as good a pediatrician-parent team as anyone could find.

I find it ironic that in emergencies—when it is so serious that it may be a life or death situation for your child—you don't get to choose the emergency doctor the way you choose your pediatrician. We were lucky we lived in a small town where we knew most of the physicians on call. Often people aren't that lucky. Usually, you must simply work with whoever is in charge in the best way you can. If it is nighttime, you may get a total stranger who has just got out of bed, or worse yet, someone who has been up handling emergency cases for the last twenty-four hours. You are panicked and confused. Your mind is racing a million miles an hour with the worst of thoughts. How do you hand your precious child, who desperately needs you now more than ever, over to a total stranger and trust that he or she knows what's best for your child? You don't. You hand your child over, but you don't back off. In fact, you assert yourself, if necessary, to stay involved. We did, and our son is alive today because we did.

HE MOVED FROM PARK INTO DRIVE, BUT WAS STILL IN LOW GEAR

I'm not sure what made me call back and beg to have Karen meet us at the hospital that horrible morning. I knew Alex was very sick, but I didn't realize he was so close to death. I guess we had learned the hard way how to handle a crisis situation. Our first medical crisis with Alex occurred when he was seventeen months old and I was eight-plus months pregnant with Marty. We were living in Brooklyn, New York, at the time, only five blocks from a community hospital, but the experience was a total disaster.

Alex woke us up at 5:00 A.M. crying. It was Saturday morning, so we put him in the bed between us and tried to go back to sleep. About an hour later, he woke me up shaking. At first I thought he was having a bad dream. I tried to comfort him, but it didn't help. When I realized something was wrong, I tried unsuccessfully to arouse him. I shook Tom awake, and he flipped on the light. Alex's skin was pale and bluish. I grabbed Alex by the torso under his arms and held him up. He stopped shaking, but his head flopped over to the side and he went totally limp. A stream of saliva dribbled down his face, and I thought he was dying. We were pretty sure it was a seizure, but never having seen one before, we were just guessing. What was particularly confusing was that we thought seizures were harmless neural events. This certainly didn't look harmless. While Tom threw on his clothes, I remember trying to keep Alex conscious. "Come on, big guy. Stick with me, big guy.

It's your mommy. You're going to be okay. I love you, big guy."
Nonetheless, he seemed to move in and out of consciousness. We
made a quick decision to get him to the hospital ourselves. Tom
threw a blanket over Alex and ran out into the cold with him. I
stayed back to call our pediatrician. Besides, I was in no shape to
run down icy streets, since I was as pregnant as a tank.

It had snowed several inches the day before and the sidewalks
were a mess, so Tom ran right down the middle of the deserted
early morning street. About a block from the hospital, a cop pulled
alongside Tom and asked if there was a problem. Tom jerked his
head "yes" but didn't slow down. The police car sped ahead to warn
the ER staff that there was a guy tearing down the street with a sick
child. Tom was greeted by a doctor who ushered him into an examination room. Breathlessly Tom tried to explain that there was
something wrong with Alex, that he thought he had had a seizure.
Alex's face was no longer bluish, but he was pale, vacant, and unable to sit up in Tom's lap.

"Well, he seems all right now," the physician said calmly, beginning to slowly, very slowly, ask questions like, "Has he been sick?"

"What do you mean, 'He seems all right'?" Tom said incredulously as he became more insistent. "There is something *wrong*
with him. This *isn't* normal."

As if on cue, Alex started to go into another seizure. Tom had
been in the ER nearly ten minutes. At this point, he recalls that
the guy began to shift from park into drive. But he was still very
much in low gear. At least he had the sense to summon another
more senior doctor. A nurse was called in to assist, but still there
was no sense of urgency. Meanwhile, I had called our pediatrician,
who couldn't do anything except to say, "Call me again when you
get to the emergency room." Despite the fact that we had given a
lot of thought to choosing a well-regarded pediatrician in Manhat-
tan, he had no privileges at the hospital in Brooklyn. Unlike our
current situation with Karen, there were many hospitals, each with
a different medical staff. He could give us comforting advice, he

could try to talk to the staff at the Brooklyn hospital, but that was about all he could do. I waddled down the icy sidewalk as fast as I could, being extra careful to pick my way over the icy footprints and ridges. The last thing we needed right then was for me to fall and go into premature labor.

I worried all of the way to the hospital. My only experience with this emergency room had been more than disturbing. Two years before, I had been jogging along a path in Prospect Park when I slipped on a rock and nearly broke my ankle. I limped into the emergency room, which was a block away. They X-rayed my ankle, found it wasn't broken, but had to cast it because I had severely torn some ligaments. To my horror, the doctor who put on my cast was noticeably drunk. Enclosed in a small examination room with him, I became nauseous from the overpowering smell of stale alcohol and cigarettes on his breath. Now here I was with my son, my seventeen-month-old helpless baby, in exactly the same emergency room. While I was willing to risk the marginal quality of the physicians myself, I wanted my son out of that hospital in the worst way.

I arrived at the hospital just as they were drawing Alex's blood. We winced as we watched them poke him repeatedly trying to hit a vein. Twenty minutes had gone by and Alex was still seizing, lying stiffly on the table in a fetal position, unconscious and shaking. We watched a slow parade of technicians move in and out of the room, wheeling in a chest X-ray machine, scribbling notes on a pad, and taking Alex's pulse for the umpteenth time. Tom was having a tough time restraining me, for I was hysterically quizzing every physician in sight as to what was going on and what they were going to do. It wasn't until the blood work came back several minutes later that anyone reacted with a sense of emergency. His blood gas levels were alarming, meaning that he was breathing, but not enough oxygen was reaching his brain. Suddenly, we were backed out of the room as an entire team of doctors converged on Alex. His condition was now critical.

Things began happening. An IV needle was put into his wrist, an oxygen mask was strapped over his face, and he was hooked up to heart rate, blood pressure, and oxygenation monitors. They started pumping huge doses of Valium and phenobarbital into him. Within minutes, his seizure stopped and they began to stabilize him. I remember accompanying Alex to the pediatric ICU not long afterward. His face was nearly as white as the hospital sheet, save a few bright red blotches on his cheeks. Tom walked on one side of his stretcher holding his limp hand, and I was on the other. The nurse in charge was wheeling him through the halls, shooing people out of the way, yelling, "Let us through, please; we've got a very sick baby here." Indeed we had.

Despite its poor beginnings, our experience in the Brooklyn hospital turned out all right for Alex. After reaching the emergency room and trying to comprehend what was going on, I called our pediatrician. He asked to speak with the physician in charge. Despite the fact that the emergency team was slow to respond to Alex's condition, our pediatrician felt that they were now doing all of the right things to stabilize him. I relaxed a little and let go of my "it's us against them" mentality. By the time we reached the pediatric ICU, I was a human being again and willing to work with the staff, if for no other reason, for Alex's sake. After spending several nights in the ICU, Alex was released.

We know a lot more now than we did then:

We've learned that not everyone in an emergency room knows how to handle a pediatric case. We've learned that in an inner-city hospital, and perhaps elsewhere, you may be competing with gunshot wounds, stabbing victims, and the like. And, we know it may be hard to get their attention if your child is not dripping blood.

We now recognize the importance of being calm. In retrospect, I wonder if the doctors might have listened to me had I not been hysterical.

We know how important it is to get the attention of the emergency physicians and provide them with the critical facts. Maybe if we had got that information across sooner, everyone would have responded with a greater sense of urgency.

We've learned to trust our intuition and in turn to develop a sense of trust when the right person is treating our child. If we don't feel that we can trust that person, we must do whatever we can, as sensitively as possible, to see that our child gets the proper attention from someone else:

> *First*, we ask to speak to the director of the emergency room to discuss the care of our child.
>
> *Second*, we discuss the possibility (or risks) of transferring him elsewhere.
>
> *Third*, we ask someone medically knowledgeable, like our family physician or pediatrician, to intervene on our behalf. In the end, that is what we had to do.

LETTING GO OF THE BALL

I've never been a great team player, and giving up control has always been hard for me, as was so painfully evident in that emergency room. As a thirteen-year-old, I was tall and gawky, with long legs, spindly arms, and an incredible reach. In theory, I made a better basketball player than a ballerina, so I tried out for the women's junior varsity and made the team. I must confess that I spent a good deal of the season on the bench, and it was my first and last year on the basketball team. It wasn't because I was the worst person on the team; I wasn't by far. Nor was it because we lost three times as many games as we won. It was because I had a dilemma—I just couldn't figure when to let go of the ball.

When the ball was passed to me, I'd waste no time dribbling toward the basket. But just when I was within shooting distance, I'd experience a momentary pang of confusion. Should I go for the basket myself or pass it to a teammate closer to the basket who may or may not miss? In that flash of indecision, I'd blow the whole moment by not trusting her—I'd either shoot too late or pass the ball too late. To this day, I have a hard time letting go of the ball when it comes to Alex's medical care. It has taken me a long time to realize that far more good can be accomplished with a team approach, even if it means that sometimes I don't control the process as much as I would like.

It's Not Always Like the Movies

Sometimes in a crisis, you are asked, or forced, to step aside for a while, particularly if drastic life-saving procedures are required. It's the turning point where most parents either set the stage to become a part of the healing team or else back off in retreat. It was during Alex's second hospitalization of his life, when he was nearly two, that we learned the hard way how to stay involved.

After experiencing his first prolonged seizure at seventeen months of age, Alex was put on Dilantin, a long-term antiseizure medication. It was a terrible thing to have to do to a toddler who had begun walking just months before. He was too young to tell us what he was feeling, but we read the side effects on the package insert and were horrified: *ataxia, slurred speech, decreased coordination, dizziness, and mental confusion.* We wondered how he would ever develop normally, viewing the world through a cloud of medication. When he went seizure-free for six months, we consulted with the neurologist again and jointly decided to taper the medication over time and see how he did. The effects were dramatic—it was as if he had stepped out of a dense fog into the bright sunlight. It was the Alex we had once known, only now he was nearly a year older.

Our euphoria didn't last long, though, for three weeks after we eliminated the medication, he had a second massive seizure.

We were visiting my brother's family in rural Virginia for Thanksgiving when Alex had his second seizure. Once again, Alex woke up early, went back to sleep in our bed, and woke up seizing uncontrollably. But this time, we were in a strange place, forty-five minutes from a country hospital. Luckily, my brother's neighbor was an emergency medical technician, who was able to get an IV in Alex and get him to the hospital by ambulance. Even so, he was still seizing when they arrived at the hospital. It was early in the morning, the day after Thanksgiving, and their emergency room staff just wasn't prepared for a pediatric case like Alex's. We tried to call our neurologist in New York, who quickly became our ex-neurologist because he did not believe in having an answering service—he was nowhere to be found. No one in the emergency room seemed to know quite what to do. Having learned from our earlier experience, Tom and I explained the circumstances and calmly tried to tell them what we thought they *should* do.

The first thing they did was shoo Tom and me out of the emergency room and tell us to sit in the waiting room. Nearly an hour went by, and we heard nothing. Getting very anxious over what was happening, we walked into the emergency room area. The physician in charge was furious and had a receptionist escort us back to the waiting room. She literally locked the door between the waiting room and the ER! By this time, my brother, who was waiting with us, had called his friend, a local pediatrician who had privileges at the hospital, and asked him to come to the hospital to see if he could help. Nearly thirty minutes went by—nothing. We thought about the situation and decided it was not right. We understood that they might not want us underfoot, but we had a right to know what was going on. So, we staged our own scene right out of the movie *Kramer vs. Kramer*.

In *Kramer vs. Kramer*, Dustin Hoffman's son is injured on the playground and has to go to an emergency room. When the physician tells Hoffman his son will need some stitches and requests that he wait outside, Hoffman forcefully insists he is going to be with him "because he's my son." We decided that Tom, the calmer one of the two of us, would play Hoffman's role. We had reached a critical point in the rural hospital where we knew we had to intervene, if not for Alex's sake, then for our own feelings of helplessness and inadequacy as parents. Tom went to the receptionist and asked to speak to the head of the emergency room staff—immediately. He calmly told him that we wanted to be near Alex and to see what was going on. He reassured him that we would not interfere or become hysterical parents, but he was quite insistent that they had no right to prevent us from being at Alex's side—he was *our* son.

It worked, but unfortunately it didn't play out as neatly as in the movies. Alex's seizure lasted for nearly three hours—it was a devastating neurological insult that never should have happened (we later learned that he could have been put under general anesthesia early on to stop the seizure). Once stabilized, he was airlifted to the University of Virginia's hospital. Tom rode with Alex and didn't leave his side until a knowledgeable pediatric neurologist got involved in his case.

The Perfect Team

Alex's bout with the *E. coli* bug at four years of age was the third hospitalization of his life. His condition was so critical, with so little room for error, that it was fortunate Tom and I were finally able to work with his medical personnel as a team. Sometimes we had our doubts, but it always worked out in the end. I'll never forget our first evening at Children's Hospital in Boston. Two critical care physicians ushered us into a small conference room for our first discussion of Alex's condition. They were both well dressed and all business. The more senior of the two introduced himself and his colleague, and then instead of saying, "How are you guys doing?" or something comforting like, "Alex had a rough trip here but is resting comfortably now," he began the meeting with, "So, how much do you want done for your son?" The shock of that statement dissolved any hope I had for Alex's recovery in an instant like an atomic explosion. It was a scene right out of my former career in business—sitting in a smartly appointed conference room, backed up against the wall, wrangling over a deal. But this wasn't some business deal we were discussing, this was my son, and nothing else at that moment meant anything more to me than him. The room was suddenly very stuffy. I looked over at Tom and I might as well have been sitting next to a ghost; his face was so drained of color that his eyes seemed like black, hollow indentations.

Without even thinking, I shot back, "Are you telling me he is going to die?" "Probably," the physician answered, and then with an incredible emotional charge in the air, we discussed Alex's case, the odds of his recovery, and what would most likely happen over the next twenty-four hours. The conversation went on for two hours. By the end of it, I accepted for the first time since the onset of his illness that Alex probably was not going to make it. But I also vowed I wouldn't give up without a fight, and they made a commitment to help us in any way they could. They reassured us he was in the best possible place—that a superb team of physicians would be working with Alex. Their businesslike approach had been hard to take, but by the end of the conversation, I was convinced we were dealing with intelligent, skilled, and compassionate physicians. They reassured us that we would meet all of the team members in the morning and told us to try to get some sleep. Right. Tom and I stayed up most of the night discussing our deepest fears. It was not a conversation of much hope.

Alex's medical team was huge. Although we were in the ICU early, it looked like they were giving out free coffee and doughnuts at Alex's bedside, for there were so many people crowded around us. One by one, they introduced themselves using their first names:

the attending physicians, the residents, the interns, the kidney specialist, the neurologist, the surgeon, the respiratory therapist, the physical therapist, the dialysis support team, and the blood banker.

"Hi, I'm Jed, the blood banker," he said. "I'm the physician in charge of all the blood products your son will be receiving."

"Yeah, I used to be a blood banker, too," I said, trying a little black humor, "but I did it on Wall Street."

He laughed politely, not quite knowing what to say in return. He turned out to be one of our best sources of emotional support throughout Alex's entire illness. We could always count on Jed to be honest and direct—he brought us good news and bad news, and he was always there for us.

Without really thinking about it, we successfully passed the ball to the other team members. We didn't feel alone in fighting for Alex's life. Nor did we feel helpless or that we had lost control. We knew it was going to take a lot—maybe a miracle—to make him well. We knew we had to manage the team to Alex's best advantage. Oddly enough, I found myself falling back on the old management adage I had learned in business: Managing is all about *planning, controlling, and organizing.*

We never began a day without asking for the day's *plan*. In the early days of his illness, the plan for his treatment changed practically every hour as his condition shifted, but every action was patiently explained to us. By our presence and questions, we were included in the decision-making process, which gave us a feeling of *control* over the situation. Once the team became more familiar with us and we with them, we found a few team members who would unselfishly let us vent our fears, frustrations, and hopes on them. It was in talking with one soft-spoken, unbelievably calm, and exceptionally bright resident named John that we were able to get a handle on all that was happening. He did a lot to help us *organize* our thoughts, our feelings, and our approach to Alex's healing process. In many ways, John represented the entire spirit of Alex's medical team.

CREATING A POSITIVE HEALING ENVIRONMENT

What can you do to help create a positive healing environment for your child in which everyone is working together as a team?

Always ask whether the person is aware of your child's condition and medical history when meeting a team member for the first time. Never get into a discussion with a medical person who has not taken the time to understand your child's case. If the individual has not reviewed your child's records, he or she will typically ask you to give a brief summary of your understanding of your child's illness or injury, any special concerns, etc.

Recognize and understand your emotions while observing the reactions of team members. Emotions are not weaknesses, and it is appropriate to express your feelings and emotions in discussions with team members as long as they don't get in the way of factual discussions. In fact, it is shared feelings that often draw a team together.

Don't be afraid to openly express your fears or your concerns. Doctors are people, too. Let them know your philosophy on life support, blood transfusions, extraordinary life-saving methods, and so forth. If you are uncomfortable or have a difficult time discussing these issues, ask to speak with the hospital chaplain. The chaplain will be an objective sounding board to help you sort out your feelings. He or she also can join your discussions with medical personnel or can act as a go-between for you and your medical team.

Try to phrase your opinions as questions. This will permit a two-way dialogue and will give you a sense of whether you are being heard. For example, your child may be in pain, and you might suspect that the pain medication levels are too low. You could approach the situation in one of two ways:

DIRECTLY: "My child is in pain. She needs more medication."

AS A QUESTION: "Do my daughter's grimaces mean that she is still in pain despite the medication?"

Either approach *might* work, but by using the second approach—asking a question—you enlist the doctor's support in making the decision without putting him or her on the defensive.

Have conversations in settings that are comfortable to you. Some parents are comfortable having conversations in front of their children. Others are not. Some need to have discussions in private in order to be able to focus. Others will willingly talk in a room full of people. Before engaging in a serious discussion, ask yourself if you feel stressed by the environment. If so, try to change the environment. We often found that it was far better to have serious discussions with Alex's medical team outside the ICU. We didn't like to talk in front of Alex, even if he was sleeping, and the high level of noise and activity was distracting for both us and the physicians.

Try your best to understand the thinking of a team member if you do not agree with him or her. Put yourself in his or her situation. Don't be afraid to ask, "Why?" or to request additional explanations. Be flexible, be open to fresh perspectives, and above all else, be reasonable.

WE'RE NOT DOCTORS, WE'RE PARENTS, AND JUST AS IMPORTANT

We learned a lot in the process of Alex's illness about trust and about being team players, not just spectators. We asked them to care for our son as if he were their own child, and they did. We learned a lot about communicating effectively with the rest of the team, and we tried never to let ourselves be intimidated by people more knowledgeable than us. We did that by adopting an attitude that it was *their job not only to heal our son, but also to help us be more effective parents—to help us heal as well.* We didn't let up until we were sure we understood what was going on and what, if anything, they could do for our son. We asked very direct questions and got very direct answers. We asked them to describe complex procedures in layperson's terms. Sometimes we asked them to explain something four times before we finally "got it." We didn't allow ourselves to be defensive or embarrassed by our lack of understanding—*after all, we're not doctors, we're parents, and we're just as important.*

5

PARENTS ARE
PRIMARY

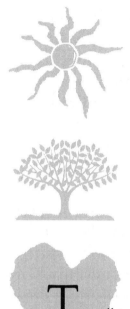

Try walking through the hall of the pediatric floor of most any hospital. Look at the young children sitting alone in high chairs. Watch those scooting around behind the nurse's station in walkers, banging into nurses' and doctors' knees trying to attract some attention. Look in on older children, mindlessly channel-surfing alone in their rooms. Watch a child's face brighten as you or anyone approaches, and it will leave you with no question about how important you are to your child's healing and recovery. We live in a high-tech world of miracle medicine—I know, I've seen nearly all there is to offer. We can cure most anything, but there is no question in my mind that *the real healing of children begins with the parents.*

Of all the people milling around a pediatric floor, children can instantly spot a parent. I've spent so much time on pediatric floors with my son that sometimes I feel like Saint Francis of Assisi. All I have to do is hang out with my son in the playroom and the other children come flocking. Brittany wants to show me the kitten she's painted, William wants me to read him a story, and Stephanie crawls into my lap and just wants to sit and be held. I resist the urge to ask them, "Where *is* your mother? Where *is* your father?" Cory, a twenty-month-old boy with tennis-ball fuzz for hair and dusty-gray eyes, was one of the most memorable ones. He was hospitalized with high fever and infection and was waiting to have a new shunt planted in his brain. His sense of balance was off, so he careened around the floor in a walker like a whirling dervish. During the two weeks his stay overlapped ours, his grandmother visited occasionally. I saw his mother only once.

If the nurses left Cory alone in his room, he screamed nonstop for hours. So the nurses let him scoot around the floor, hoping that parents, visitors, and other children would entertain him. The strategy worked great until he met me. A perceptive young guy, he noticed I was always there with Alex, playing with him, assisting him on art projects, or just rocking him. One day he dropped a squeeze toy he was toting around and let out a whimper. I went over to Cory, picked up the toy, and smiled as I handed it back. I looked into his deep, sad eyes, and that was it. Thereafter he screamed for my attention every time he saw me. *All I had done was pick up his toy and smile.* He'd be scooting around, talking to anyone who would listen, and then he'd spot me walking across the floor and let out a blood-curdling *eeeeeeeEEEEEEEE*. The nurses couldn't figure out what was bothering him, but I knew. I tried to steer clear of him for the remainder of his stay unless I was prepared to entertain him. I wanted to help him and make him feel better, but it was never enough. What he really needed was his mother. I didn't want him to become attached to me and have to suffer the loss of *two* mothers!

Nurses Are Great, but They Are Not Parents

Children need their parents even more when they are not feeling well, particularly if they are hospitalized. They must sleep in a strange bed, in a place teeming with pungent, antiseptic smells and confusing, scary noises. No one is familiar to them. Most people are just faces—faces that peer in at them, bend over them, prod them, poke them, and often inflict pain.

Too many parents assume their children are well taken care of in a hospital. They are, sort of. But, there is no way they get the same amount of attention and comfort they receive at home. Nurses are not baby-sitters, they're nurses, many of whom are mothers or fathers of young children themselves. They care, but they are harried, often shuttling between four to six children at once. They draw up medications, check temperatures, clean up disasters, and tote teddy bears, but they are not baby-sitters. When they have the time, they are more than willing to comfort your child or rock him or her to sleep. But they can only give your child undivided attention after every other child has been given medication, after any emergencies have been re-solved, and after all their patients are settled. They don't resent parents who want to help with their child's care. On the contrary, they encourage it—it makes their job easier, and they know children get better sooner when a parent is there to comfort them.

Jill was a pediatric nurse about our age, whom we met during Alex's long stay in Boston. On the surface, she was caring, orga-nized, and rather businesslike. But on the inside, Jill was a saint. She tried to treat every patient as if it were her own child. At the same time, she recognized that her job was to care for many chil-dren at once. She cared for Alex at nights following his transfer from the ICU to the medical floor. She knew it was a miracle he was still alive; she knew what we had been through, and she would do almost anything to support us.

It was 11:30 one night, long past Alex's normal bedtime, and he just wouldn't settle down and go to sleep. He had been going through withdrawal from pain medications since leaving the ICU. His days were spent flailing around in agitation. He cried and moaned nearly all of the time, and he could barely raise his head. He was far, very far, from being able to entertain himself. Neither Tom nor I could spend more than two hours at a time with him without practically moaning and crying ourselves. The nights were the only relief we got, so when he wouldn't go to sleep, it was a major crisis. That night Tom was determined not to leave him until he was asleep. Jill stopped by to see how Alex was doing and saw the exhaustion and anguish on Tom's face. She told Tom not to worry, that she would be finished with her rounds soon and would stay with Alex as long as he needed. In a few minutes, she returned as promised with an armful of books.

"Go," she said. "Go back to the hotel and get some sleep." She looked at our son, who was pitifully flip-flopping back and forth and moaning. Practically in tears herself, she said, "Get some sleep—you're going to need the strength for tomorrow." She wasn't kidding.

The next morning, she told us Alex had fallen asleep almost immediately in her lap in a rocking chair. It was as if he didn't want his dad to leave him unless he knew that someone else loving would be there. Jill was that person, and as a nurse, she's more an exception than the rule. When I think about the situation, it was 11:30 at night. It had taken Jill over three hours to get her other patients settled and to sleep. Had we not been there, Alex would have cried alone in his room for hours. No matter how much she cared for Alex, and ultimately for us, she had a job to do—he wasn't her only patient.

Jill went out of her way for *us*, not just our son, and I think there is a real message in that. You might think that nurses spend more time comforting children whose parents are absent, but I've observed the opposite to be true. More often than not, nurses seem to be more attentive to patients whose parents are visible. It is sort of an attitude like, "If you care, then I care." Volunteers also spend a great deal of time on a pediatric floor relieving tired or hungry parents, more so it would seem than comforting children who are alone.

As a parent, on some level I wish you could see what I've seen, although in reality I wouldn't want to wish it on anyone. I've lain awake nearly all night beside my son in the hospital listening to a tiny baby girl cry and hack away with a croupy cough. No one sat up with her and held her the way her mother would. I've walked around a pediatric floor at 3:00, 4:00, and 5:00 A.M. and felt the loneliness of the place creep up around me and make me shudder. I've seen children waiting all day for their parents to come visit, and I've seen and felt their disappointment at being let down. I've had a lot of kids so desperate for their mothers that they clung to me and wouldn't let go. Jill summed up the view that I think many nurses have about parents:

> Of course it makes an incredible difference to a child to have a parent with them. It's so obvious they get well lots faster. Some parents just park their sick kids here, and we never see them again until they come to take their child home. I can't tell those parents what to do. I'm not their mother . . . nor can I be a mother to their child. That's not my role.

IF AND WHEN YOU CAN'T BE THERE

I don't want you to think that you have to sit beside your child's bed around-the-clock to comfort your child. That is not the message at all. In my son's case, I think I was there for me as much as I was for him. We *both* had a lot of healing to do. His near-death experience was so chilling and so disturbing that I was afraid to let him out of my sight. I had come so close to losing him that I wanted to be involved in every aspect of his care and recovery. I also had the flexibility to spend a great deal of time with him, which is not true for many parents. No one can tell you the "right" amount of time to spend with your child. That is something only you know. Just as I did, you have to decide what works for *both* you and your child. One thing I'm sure of, though, is that you can never err by spending too much time with your child.

Like any other aspect of parenting, it's the quality of the time you give your child that counts. A bouncy redheaded three-year-old girl roomed next to us for a while. For whatever reason, her mother could not visit every day. But never a day went by that she didn't call her daughter on the phone and talk for nearly an hour. Her mother would call the front desk and have the call transferred to her daughter's room, where a nurse would answer and hand the phone to the little girl in her crib. You could overhear the little girl in the hall chattering on and on about her teddy bear, her pajamas, her doll, and making up stories. We all thought it was hysterical, but it worked; she was a happy, content patient for her five-day stay. Even though her mother was not always at her side, she knew that her mother cared, and her mother knew that she was content.

If you cannot be with your hospitalized child as much as you want, don't make things worse for yourself by feeling guilty. You may have other children who need your attention just as much, or getting time off from your job may be impossible. The mother in the preceding story was able to comfort her child without being present. It was obvious in that little girl's behavior that she was receiving warm and caring support from her mother. An hour or so on the phone with her mother was all she needed to feel secure. A similar approach may work for your child as well.

However you manage your child's hospitalization, I don't think you can ever underestimate how frightening being left alone in a hospital can be. I know that Alex would never have adjusted to being left alone for a significant amount of time. For one thing, he was so debilitated by his illness that he was not physically capable of getting around and watching out for himself. He also had a tremendous fear of being alone and was terrified by anyone who even resembled a doctor.

What do you do if your child is like Alex, and you can't spend the time with your child that he or she needs to heal?

Call your child frequently if he or she is able or old enough to talk on the phone. It will be important for your child to know that you are thinking about him or her.

Talk to your child's primary nurse about your concerns over leaving your child alone in the hospital. Ask him or her to help you do everything possible to see that caring people are with your child as much as possible. Most nurses I've encountered would take a request like that very seriously.

Arrange for family members and friends to stay with your child when you cannot. When your child is hospitalized, many people will offer to help in any way they can. Sitting with your child is a tangible way in which they can be of tremendous support.

Ask the social worker to have the hospital chaplain visit your child on a regular basis. The social worker might also be able to organize a team of volunteers to sit with your child, read to your child, or take your child for walks around the hospital.

Even though you are not at your child's bedside, stay on top of his or her medical care. Call the hospital several times a day and ask to speak with your child's nurse, physicians, or the resident physician on duty. Ask very specific questions about how your child is doing, including how your child's recovery is progressing and how he or she is eating, sleeping, and emotionally coping with the situation.

Once you show how concerned you are about your child's well-being, nurses, doctors, volunteers, family, and friends will go out of their way to help you. People who have the time want to help— they just have to know how.

WHO WILL ANSWER THE QUESTIONS IF NOT YOU?

In the beginning I had a very hard time dealing with Alex's illness. Never a day went by that I didn't wonder why such bad things had to happen to me and my family. I knew it wasn't rational, but I always wondered in some way whether I was to blame—whether I had done something wrong to bring all of this evil upon us. I wondered whether Alex was really inside the body lying almost lifeless before me. I was filled with an emptiness like I had never felt before. I'd sit with Alex, holding his warm, bloated hand, trying to be strong, trying to maintain control. But inside, my mind would be screaming "WHY? WHY? WHY?" so loudly that it would make my whole body buzz. Time lost its meaning, and every sensation—what I saw, heard, smelled, and felt—had a rawness about it; I felt my soul was sitting out there all alone, totally exposed and vulnerable.

It came as quite a surprise to me to discover that Alex's younger brother, Marty, was having similar thoughts and asking similar questions. I honestly thought that he was too young to comprehend what was going on (he was two and a half at the time). How wrong I was. His line of questioning went something like this:

"Mommy, why is Alex in the hospital?"

"Mommy, why did Alex get sick?"

"Mommy, did I do something wrong?"

"Mommy, is Alex going to die?"

"Mommy, what happens when you die?"

I thought I had a good handle on what being a mother means. I thought I knew how to comfort my children and be supportive. I thought I knew how to talk to them, to foster a sense of independence and well-being. But nothing, absolutely nothing, prepared me for how to deal with the grief of a child slipping away from me and his little brother pummeling me with questions that I wish I knew the answers to myself.

To this day, Marty has never really got over his older brother's brush with death. We'll be driving down a desolate country road together when he'll suddenly start quizzing me about seat belts and car accidents. When he does that, I know it's coming: "Mommy, what happens when you die?"

It's a question he's asked over and over since his brother's illness. Answers like, "If you've led a good life, you go to heaven," have never worked for him. Our discussions have become much more involved than I ever imagined conversations with a preschooler could get. Sometimes I think that we've discussed death from every imaginable perspective.

As much as I don't like using real images (like describing heaven as the most beautiful place you could imagine, with lush vegetation, buildings with golden spires, and so forth), I found they were really necessary to make Marty feel like he understood what he was hearing. He needed so much to see what I was describing that we took out an art history book so he could look at artists' depictions of hell.

He had a very hard time accepting the concept that when you die, you go away and never come back, but your soul lives on forever. The word "forever" to someone Marty's age is the amount of time it takes to eat dinner before he or she can have dessert. We spent a long time discussing the soul and the spirit, but I was never really sure how well he understood what I was saying. In his mind, the only way he could comprehend the concept of the "soul" was to think of it interchangeably with the brain: Not long after we had our discussion of the soul, he was standing up on a reasonably high platform looking down and commented, "My soul is telling me not to jump." We also discussed graveyards and burials in minute detail ("Mommy, do they put the gravestone over your head or your belly?"). And he quizzed me at length on the connection between death, ghosts, witches, and space aliens.

One of the most difficult things I found about trying to answer Marty's questions was the questions they elicited in my own mind. Alex's illness touched him in some way I'll never fully understand. Maybe it's because it touched him in the same way it touched me.

I was lucky—if you want to call it that—that Alex was too sick to ask many questions. Interestingly enough, when he recovered, he rarely asked them either. I know from some comments he makes that he's really confused about why he got sick and why he continues to have seizures. But, we have waited and will continue to wait until he is ready to talk about it. He accepts the battle scars on his body—the long incision up his belly, the puckering scars where his ostomy bag used to be, and the not insignificant scar on his ankle where an IV failed at one of the worst moments of his illness. But he never asks questions about death or an afterlife. Perhaps it is too frightening for him to discuss, or it may be that he already knows the answer.

One of the hardest things to do is to answer your child's questions when you yourself do not have the answers. You just do the best you can. Whatever you may be thinking, your child will, too. Maybe you are more prepared than I was to tackle your child's tough questions. Maybe not, but here are a few things I've learned that may help you:

Listen carefully for the occasions when your child needs to talk. Don't try to explain things on your own. Let your child ask you in his or her own words the difficult questions he or she is facing. Before rushing to answer them, allow your child to first explore the answers on his or her own. Expect your child to ask the same questions over and over. As adults we do, why shouldn't they?

Be honest with your child. Children have a way of knowing the truth, and it is far better to hear it from you than someone else. A nurse once told the story of a two-and-a-half-year-old boy whose mother did not want him to know he was dying. Yet, he knew. In his own mind, he concocted a story about going to see Santa Claus, for it was the only way he could understand.

Reassure your child that he or she has done nothing wrong. I still must admit that I occasionally wonder whether I'm being punished for something. Your child will, too. Let your child know that sometimes things just happen.

Be tolerant of your child's anger. You have to expect your child to be angry, very angry. I still am on some level, so I expect my child to be, too. It is a natural reaction under the circumstances.

Create and build hope. Don't be afraid to hope or let your child hope for fear that your optimism will be dashed. Just try to hope in small increments, day by day. Give your child something to look forward to—a visit from someone he or she loves, the end of a treatment, or the experience of walking for the first time in days. For our son, it was getting the puppy he always wanted.

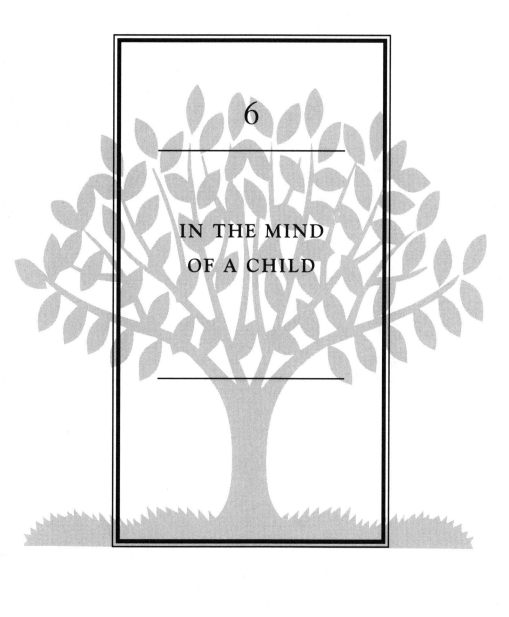

6

IN THE MIND
OF A CHILD

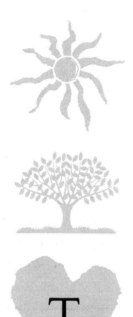

There is no question in my mind that the greatest fear of all young children is separation from their parents. It doesn't make a difference whether it hits them in a shopping mall, in a new school, or in a hospital setting. It is a paralyzing fear that can shake the confidence of the most secure child. I've learned through experience, though, that the fear of separation, like many of my children's anxieties, reflects our fears as much as theirs. And why shouldn't they feel this way? Tom and I have taught our kids to trust us. If they sense something is wrong for us, it's only natural and logical for them to be afraid as well.

The summer we moved to Vermont, some friends from New York and their three-year-old daughter came for a visit. It was a spectacularly clear day, with high white clouds, and we decided to take a chairlift ride to the summit of Mount Snow. I was holding

Alex in my lap, and Tom was sitting next to me holding Marty. Not fifty feet out of the loading platform, I realized that a chairlift ride in the winter and a chairlift ride in the summer were two very different things. Where was that nice thick blanket of snow beneath me? I had an instantaneous vision of Alex slipping out of the chair and falling down onto the rugged mountainside below us. I locked my arms around Alex and gripped the overhead bar so tightly that my knuckles were pasty yellow.

Alex was having a fine time, yelling, "Wheeeee," and kicking his legs in excitement. He had never shown a fear of heights before. Suddenly he sensed my fear and started chanting, "Get down, get down." I didn't know what to do. I tried to relax—to pretend I was having a good time—but Alex's chanting and squirming made me all the more nervous. Then the chairlift stopped and swung back and forth in the air for nearly a minute. Marty started to panic. I looked over at Tom and he did the only thing he could think of—he started singing "Wheels on the Bus" as loud as he could, and I and the kids joined in. We sang it over and over, all the way to the top.

At the top, I leaped off the chairlift, and my legs nearly buckled because I was so faint. I felt terrible for transmitting my fear to my children. When our friends stepped off the chairlift after us, I noticed that they, too, were singing with their daughter. Her dad had experienced the same fleeting panic I had, and both of her parents were emotional wrecks. We recovered in the cool air and hiked around on the summit, taking pictures and helping the kids pick fistfuls of wildflowers. Then the weather changed abruptly. The wind began to blow, the sky covered over with fast-moving clouds, and it started to sprinkle. I had avoided thinking about it, but now I had to face my fear of the inevitable trip back down.

Despite the marginal weather, I wanted to walk, but Tom felt we should take the chairlift down and try to give the kids a positive experience. He was right. The other couple vowed never to set foot on a chairlift again and spent two hours walking down in the wind and rain, carrying their daughter much of the way. Before getting back on the chairlift, I mentally prepared myself to relax by thinking about curling up in the rocking chair on the porch of my mom's oceanfront home, watching the waves roll in. Tom and I also did a lot of cheerleading on that trip down. It was as much for me as it was for them:

"Hey, guys, isn't this fun?"

"Moving chairs, stepping down . . . Wheee!"

"Wow, look over at that mountain. Can you see our house?"

Much to our amazement, the boys really did have fun. I, too, didn't think it was all that bad. Now, several years later, the kids are beginning to show an interest in skiing. Schussing down the hill with Mom and Dad is pretty good, but the real excitement is riding the chairlift to the top.

I thought a lot about our chairlift experience when Alex was in the hospital. I thought about it when we allowed Marty to see Alex in the ICU for the first time. We told him the ICU was a really cool place and it was full of neat equipment (he didn't know how neat it was—that it had saved Alex's life). We prepared him for the shock of seeing his brother all hooked up to tubes and wires by telling him that Alex would look like a space alien. When it came time to enter the ICU, we took Marty by the hand and took deep breaths. We could tell he was scared, but his response upon entering—"Hey, this place looks like fun!"—made us laugh. It also made us realize that we had one less stress to deal with—it looked as if Marty was going to be able to handle the situation okay.

I Want My Mommy, I Want My Daddy

I've thought a lot about who feels the pain of separation more—you or your young child. Young children don't worry about how sick they are. They don't worry about how long it takes to recover from an illness. What worries them most is the fear that their mommy and daddy might go away and never come back. Their fear is particularly intense when they must also be restrained. They thrash, kick, wriggle, writhe, and strain as if their life depended on it. They search the room looking for you with piercing eyes, trying to comprehend how you could abandon them under the circumstances. They try to reach out to you, and when that fails, they give up in despair. It is not the illness or injury itself that is most traumatic for your child. It's the separation from you that causes your child the greatest pain.

There were times when Alex was younger when I had to pry him off me, hand by hand, and pass his rigid and screaming body over to a doctor or nurse. There were times when he looked at me with such fear and betrayal that I questioned whether medical science was worth it. Tom and I often wondered whether we would be accused of negligence if we walked away from it all and let nature take its course. But in the end, we always did what we had to do as parents—we stayed at his side if possible, fighting back tears and calmly trying to reassure him that things would be okay.

When he had to be physically taken away from us, we built up a steel wall of control and tried to rationalize how separation hurt us more than it hurt him. We'd give him "Pongo," his favorite stuffed dog, to guard him. We'd tuck his baby blanket up next to his face and tell him that his blanket was there to hold him when we were not. Once we sent a tape of Beethoven's *Archduke Trio*, his favorite music, to surgery with him. These were only *things*, but they were things that meant something to him at the time—things that were very much a part of his world. I knew they were no substitute for Tom or me, but I hoped they would help him bridge the connection to us and give him faith that we would always be back.

At some time, all of us with children will most likely have to face dreadful and anxiety-producing experiences such as these. How do you keep them from terrifying your child for years to come? You don't—you really can't control your child's fears. But you can be aware that you, too, are a source of your child's fear. It's never easy to hide your own anxiety. It blooms on your face, resonates in your voice, chills your touch, and transforms your warm hugs into desperate clutches. Your child picks up on your fear without your even so much as uttering a word.

Whatever you do, however you manage it, you have to try your best not to add your own fears to the mountain of fears your child may already have. I know, for example, that separation hurts me a lot more than it hurts my children. I always consciously try to think about something positive and relaxing. I also try to give my children a reason to trust me by always being there for them, if not in body, in spirit:

- Assure your child that you will be thinking about him or her constantly.
- Leave your child with something (like a toy or a favorite blanket) that *both* of you know is special.
- Ask to be with your child the moment he or she awakes or returns from a procedure.
- Tell the nurse or medical assistant how to best comfort your child (e.g., through singing, massaging his or her back, or whatever).

FANTASIES AND DISTORTIONS

Sometime during the preschool years a child's intense fear of separation gives way to more complex fears. With ever-active imaginations, preschoolers tend to confuse fantasy with reality and distort things out of proportion. The couch that becomes a pirate ship and the Oriental rug that becomes a sea of sharks, octopuses, and stingrays can provide hours of entertainment. But a tiny needle that becomes a huge scary instrument of torture can terrify a preschooler beyond belief.

During the summer Alex was in Children's Hospital in Boston, we tried our best to make life for Marty as normal as possible, but it wasn't easy. Kids in wheelchairs, kids wrapped up in bandages like mummies, kids without hair, and kids with IV poles, nose tubes, and carts full of electronic equipment became more commonplace to him than healthy, active kids. He became obsessed with medicine and the human body, and although he was only two and a half years old, fancy words like "dialysis," "ostomy," and "stethoscope" crept into his vocabulary. When Alex's condition became less critical, Tom and I took turns exploring Boston with Marty. The city became a great big backyard to him.

One day, I decided to take Marty to the Museum of Science. On the subway to the museum, Marty fell asleep in the stroller. As fate would have it, he woke up in the Human Body Discovery Room. He was totally disoriented. At first, I think he thought he was back in the ICU. But he looked around and quickly figured out we were in a place with *lots* of interesting things to see and do. He was instantly drawn to a life-size human skeleton sitting on a bicycle. If you sat on the exercise cycle in front of the skeleton and pedaled, the skeleton's legs would pump up and down like yours. Marty could not get enough of this exhibit, which he called "the bone man on the bicycle." I pedaled as he sat in my lap, squealing with delight, until a line formed behind us. I only got him off the bicycle by showing him the life-size human body whose organs lit up when you pushed a button. He wanted me to show him where Alex's body "hurt" so he could push the button and look at it. We lit up the brain, the large intestines, and the kidneys and talked about each one. The trip to the museum was supposed to be a diversion, but here we were discussing body parts and sick people once again! After what seemed like hours, we finally left that room and darted among space capsules, race cars, giant insects, and the like.

Of all the exciting things in the Museum of Science, it was the skeleton that Marty chose to tell Tom about that evening. His eyes grew big and round as he described the exhibit. A year and a half later, we made our first trip back to the Science Museum since Alex's illness. Marty had forgotten much of what had happened the summer Alex got sick, but he had vivid memories of the skeleton on the bicycle. He couldn't wait to get into the museum and find the exhibit again. We bought our tickets and instantly got sidetracked by giant pendulums, dinosaur bones, and the space capsule. But when Marty remembered his mission—to find the skeleton—he insisted we go directly there. We walked into the room and I pointed to it. He looked like a child who was just given his big chocolate birthday cake without any candles.

"It doesn't look the same, Mommy," he said.

He went over and hopped up on the exercise cycle now that his legs were long enough to pedal it himself, but his heart wasn't in it. In his mind, he had created something that didn't exist.

Marty illustrated a behavior that is typical of preschoolers—he confused fantasy and reality. In his mind, the skeleton had come alive when I pedaled. In reality, he discovered it was just a big plastic skeleton, like the miniature model he keeps in his bedroom. Think about how amused you have been at times by your child's active imagination. Then place your child's mind in a medical setting and imagine how the tendency to distort things out of proportion can intensify your child's fears. Alex is "Mr. Imagination." He can take a simple line like, "Curly chased a squirrel," and transform it in a matter of microseconds in his mind into, "Curly chased a squirrel into a hole, and a fox came out, and Curly and the fox went swimming in the stream and splashed each other." His imagination is especially challenging in a medical setting.

Alex views going for an X ray as entering a Chamber of Horrors. Our typical outpatient experience involves entering a dimly lit room with big, cold, octopuslike machines. He suspiciously watches the X-ray technician cover his parent with a lead apron—a *shield*. He sees and senses the technician's hastiness to bolt out of the room when the machine is turned on. For him, an X-ray machine is not something benign, and the technician's reassurances that "it won't hurt" mean nothing to him. In his five-year-old mind, an X-ray machine is something to protect yourself against. It's a totally understandable fear.

I don't try to convince Alex that having an X ray is not going to be a frightening experience. I never, ever say, "It won't hurt," because he'll fixate on the word "hurt." I try to be relaxed about the whole thing. I tell him it is going to be an interesting experience, and I try to explain how the machine works. Often I ask the technician for a copy of an X ray so he may hold it up to the light and look at it. I ask Alex to be brave, and I comfort him with my touch and my presence. I also let him know that it will be over soon. I don't try to convince Alex that his fears are irrational. I just try to make the experience as routine as possible so that one day he may see for himself that he has distorted the situation out of proportion.

I Feel Much Better, I'll Be Good Now

I once asked our neurologist to characterize Alex's seizures on a scale of 1 to 10. I guess I was looking for some comfort in understanding how his condition compared with others. At the time, he rated them a 3 on frequency and a 10 on severity. In reality, it's kind of like predicting when Los Angeles will have its next earthquake and what magnitude it will be on the Richter scale. We know earthquakes are going to happen, but we never know when or how severe they will be. We think we can look to some clues to predict them, but it doesn't always work. And when they hit, they can be unimaginable disasters.

Last summer, Tom, Marty, and Alex were playing keep-away in the yard with Alex's dog, Curly, and his rubber bone. Tom figured out how to distract Curly while Alex and Marty sneaked up and snatched his bone. When Curly lost possession of the bone, he ran around and around in circles, which made Alex giggle so hard he couldn't stand. When they got totally worked up, Tom thought it wise to shift to a calmer activity, so they moved over to the swing. Alex was standing next to the swing, when his body suddenly became rigid. He was staring blankly. Tom asked him if he was okay, and there was no response. Tom knew that was a bad sign. He scooped him up as the seizure began to take over his body and ran into the house with him. Marty ran after them, asking, "What happened? What happened?" Tom burst in the door and yelled for me. Alex was moving in and out of consciousness, so we knew that the seizure had still not generalized.

"Can you hear me, Alex? Mommy's here," I said. No response. He was staring to the extreme left and his body was rigid.

"Take a deep breath," I said. We thought we heard a faint gasp. I put my ear to his chest and felt his heart fluttering wildly, as if it were trying to take off.

"Try to turn your head off, Alex," Tom suggested. "Switch it off like a TV set." A minute went by. Anxiously Tom and I kept asking each other whether we thought the seizure was going to pass or generalize.

Marty kept asking, "What's happening? What's happening? Is Alex having a seizure?"

"I don't know," I answered. We needed some space, so I asked Marty to go find his doctor's bag. Tom kept talking to Alex, trying to reach him. After four minutes, the brain quake stopped as suddenly as it began. Luckily, it was a mild one and no emergency measures were required. Nonetheless, Marty had his play stethoscope out, poised for action.

"Are you okay, Alex?" I asked.

"I feel much better, Mommy. I'll be good now," Alex answered, speaking as if from a far-off cave.

Then he slipped into a deep sleep typical of postseizure activity.

It was the shortest seizure Alex had ever had, probably because it never generalized. But it was also the first time he had ever been able to talk right after a seizure ended. All the tension that had been building up in me during the episode came pouring out when I heard the words, "I'll be good now."

"It's *not* your fault, Alex. You didn't do anything wrong. You really don't deserve all of this. No one does. *You didn't do anything wrong.*" I was practically pleading with him, but he was fast asleep.

We couldn't believe Alex thought he was being punished for doing something wrong. It wasn't until sometime later that we discovered it is typical for five-year-olds to blame themselves for their illnesses. When I thought about it, the notion that Alex's medical problems are due entirely to random bad luck was a hard concept for even me to grasp. It seems so illogical and unfair. What could I expect him to think? I have come to realize that Alex, like any other five-year-old, needs an answer and looks for the simplest explanation: "I hurt because I did something wrong." It takes very supportive, patient, and understanding parents to dispel these feelings. We know, because we're still trying.

PROTECTING LOVED ONES

We first met Joey at Dartmouth-Hitchcock Medical Center, during Alex's second hospitalization from the *E. coli* infection. Alex had been transferred back to Dartmouth from Children's Hospital in Boston and was spending a week for neurological follow-up and general rehabilitation. When I first saw Joey, I thought he was one of the most angelic-looking children I had ever seen. He was almost nine years old at the time. His head was hairless and shiny, reflecting back the light around him. If you looked into his eyes, you looked at a contradiction—his eyes twinkled with intensity. Marty was playing with Joey's younger sister in the hospital playroom, and

I got to talking with his mother. It was then that I realized he lived in a neighboring town in Vermont. I had read about his three-year struggle with cancer in the local newspaper. I had seen the tattered photocopy of his face taped to a donation can on the counter of the local market. I had even dumped quite a bit of spare change into that can.

For the next year, our paths crossed often. Joey was in and out of the hospital for testing and treatments, and Alex was in and out, battling the physical and neurological aftermath of his bacterial infection. We never got to know the family very well. I think we were each caught up in our own medical battles, trying to cope with a day at a time. But we did get a firsthand view of their pain and Joey's tremendous courage. The spring before his tenth birthday, Joey's cancer was declared in remission. By the late summer, the cancer had returned with a vengeance and was deemed inoperable. His goal became living until his tenth birthday in November. When the doctors advised Joey that his cancer was terminal, I was told that he asked point-blank how long he had to live and was given a very direct answer of several months. They say he cried a lot but insisted that he personally tell his brothers and sisters, almost as if he were more worried about them than himself.

Children Joey's age have a tremendous amount of compassion for their families—they seek to protect their loved ones as much as they protect themselves. They are at an age when they are becoming more independent. They still want the support of their families and to know their families are there to protect them. Although Joey's behavior was typical of his age, he showed an unusual compassion for others and an incredible sensitivity to the pain his illness caused. It is said that when a child is sick, the whole family feels it. In Joey's case, the whole community felt it. He radiated love in every way—he took great care to protect his teacher and his classmates from their pain, he persevered on the gymnastics team despite debilitating chemotherapy and radiation treatments, and he appeared in a promotional videotape with Michael J. Fox to benefit David's House, a home away from home for families of children in Dartmouth-Hitchcock Medical Center. Joey didn't quite make it to his tenth birthday, but on his birthday, his fourth-grade classmates went to his grave and sent up tons of balloons with messages on them like: "Star, my horse, misses you very much (I can tell)" and "The fort we built by the river got knocked down." One message said, "Your family is doing well." Of all the messages, I'm sure that was the one he wanted to hear the most.

I Want to Make My Own Decision

In the winter, I sometimes tutor at the Alpine Academy at Mount Snow. Junior high and high school kids come from around the northeast to train as downhill ski racers. They are tutored on a one-to-one basis for their academic studies by people like me. The tutors are an interesting, somewhat ragtag, highly educated lot. We all do something else for a living, but are drawn to the mountain by the skiing, the informality of the teaching job, and the source of extra income. I tutor alongside an accountant teaching classics, a veterinarian teaching dissection, and a writer teaching *Hamlet*. One of my colleagues, Michael, is a graduate of the Great Books program at Saint John's College. He works the graveyard shift at the Retreat, a drug and rehabilitation facility in Brattleboro, as a residential adviser. A philosophical sort of fellow, I can always count on Michael to have an interesting perspective, no matter what the topic.

Last winter, Michael and I were chatting about Alex's seizure disorder. I had missed a bit of work. Everyone knew that Alex was in the hospital and that I was commuting two hours from Dartmouth. Michael told me about a friend of his, a woman in her forties who had contracted a tropical disease while living in Saigon twenty years earlier. She was later diagnosed with a life-threatening seizure disorder like Alex's. Once a professional dancer, she had given it up because the antiseizure medication affected her coordination and sense of balance. I told him how we suspected this was the case with Alex—that he was often shaky, ran a bit like an inexperienced cross-country skier, and sometimes had periods of fogginess and confusion. Michael told me that one day this woman decided she had had enough—she decided to discontinue the medication, whatever the consequences. Then she moved from western Massachusetts to Maine and started a dance school. She had been living and teaching in Maine for about four years when she told Michael that she had never been happier—she felt terrific, her dancing had improved, and she had built a highly successful dance school. Then one night not long after, she went to sleep, had a seizure, and never woke up.

I found the story really creepy, almost as if I knew the woman myself and was hearing about her death for the first time. I hadn't really thought about Alex being on long-term medication until the E. coli infection changed the nature of his seizure disorder. Since then, I had often thought about the day Alex would question whether he wanted to take his medication. But until I had that conversation with Michael, I don't think I had ever discussed it with anyone else. Michael and I were sitting in the main academic tutorial room. All around us were healthy, rosy-cheeked young skiers, and we were sitting there having an intense discussion about making life-and-death choices. In my heart, I had to admit that I thought I would have done the same thing as the dancer—I, too, would have chosen living over simply being. But it is always so easy to say what you might do when it's not really you. Michael asked me whether I thought I would try to prevent Alex from making the same decision. I just didn't know the answer.

Not all that long ago, Billy Best, a sixteen-year-old with Hodgkin's disease, made all of the national newspapers. After completing his initial treatments for cancer, he was told he needed four more months of chemotherapy and radiation. He sold some of his belongings to raise cash, packed a duffel bag, took his skateboard, and ran away. The note he left behind in his bedroom said it all: "I feel like the medicine is killing me instead of helping me."

I read the articles about Billy Best with such passion that I might well have been substituting the name "Alex" for "Billy." It frightened me to find myself taking Billy's side, not his parents', while everyone else in the country seemed to be telling Billy to go home. Maybe it's because we've seen Alex endure such pain and discomfort. Maybe it's because we've seen him knocked down again and again. Maybe it's because we've seen him struggling to be like every other kid and not quite making it. Maybe it's because we've seen him crying inconsolably with frustration. We give Alex all the support and optimism we can. But we hover over him, unable for medical reasons to let him be as independent as other kids his age. We have no idea what kind of person that will make him at age sixteen. Right now he needs both us and his medication to survive. Someday, he will no longer be the little child we can spoon-feed medicine. Then what?

CHILDREN FIRST AND PATIENTS SECOND

I think it's important to recognize that *children are children first and patients second*. This is something we grapple with every day with Alex, but it is particularly true for teenagers like Billy Best. As patients, they have the same concerns over appearance, social acceptance, and independence as any teenager. In most states, children fourteen years old or older can obtain medical treatment without parental approval as long as they demonstrate they understand the risks and benefits of the treatment. But when it comes to their ability to refuse treatment, we question their understanding and their judgment. Luckily, in most cases, you don't have to deal with these extremes. But there is a lot you can do to make sure that your child participates in the decisions concerning his or her illness.

Take the time to explain the details of what is happening to your child and try to give him or her some control over the situation. Jordan, for example, was a four-year-old with an uncontrollable seizure disorder we met in Children's Hospital. Before getting sick, he had been a child model, and it was pretty obvious why. He had a dark complexion, with big brown wide-set eyes and thick eyelashes he could practically trip on. He had undergone neurosurgery right before we met him to implant temporary electrodes in his brain for monitoring. His head was wrapped in gauze, and he looked like a miniature sheikh. For most of the day, he was confined to his room so his actions could be monitored on videotape. He was about as angry and miserable as a four-year-old could be.

It wasn't too long before his mother was miserable, too. That's how she met us. Every day, she would pull Jordan in a wagon through the halls for a few minutes of sanity. We'd also be out walking the halls—with Alex propped up with all his medical equipment in a "go-cart" (a stretcherlike vehicle with wheelchair wheels) and Marty riding shotgun on the front. We'd do laps in the hall together and then retreat to our respective rooms to endure several more hours of moaning. When Jordan's mom could no longer take it, she talked to the social worker and decided that what Jordan needed was a greater sense of control over his situation. She then did something ingenious. She went out and bought a hospital T-shirt and posted it on a board near the door. Before anyone new could enter the room or touch Jordan, he or she was accosted by Jordan, who would insist that the person sign his T-shirt. In effect, Jordan was permitted to give his "approval" for all that was done to him. It was amazing how quickly his attitude improved. It wasn't long before he and Marty were pulling each other in the wagon down the hall.

Ask for your child's opinion, and give him or her some options. It wasn't until Billy Best ran away from the prospect of four more months of chemotherapy and radiation treatments, that his physician offered him a more palatable option. Talking to Billy through the national media, he suggested that Billy could just have radiation treatments or that he could cut back on chemotherapy. What Billy did was significant—he demonstrated to all the parents of the world what can happen when an adolescent feels he no longer has control over his body, his illness, and his very being.

It's Never Easy to Reach Them

One of the hardest things we find in dealing with Alex and his illness is understanding what he is really thinking. Sometimes he talks a little about it, but most of the time we have to try to imagine what might be going on in the mind of a young child. We want to be the best possible parents for him, but often, we're just not sure what we're parenting. I've talked of some major issues confronting the parents of ill or injured children: the trauma of separation, the tendency to distort things out of proportion, the pain of realizing that children blame themselves for their sickness, the beauty of how young adolescents care about the feelings of others, and the tough choices that come with increasing independence.

Often we wonder what life would have been like had Alex not had medical problems. How would he be different? I'm sure we would still be dealing with all of the above issues; they just seem far more intense when viewed through the lens of a life-threatening medical condition. Like any other parents, we will raise our children to make informed choices, to be self-sufficient, and to care about the welfare of others. I'm sure we will make mistakes, just like anyone else. As parents of a child with a medical condition, though, we have an additional responsibility—to best prepare Alex for the day when he will manage his illness on his own.

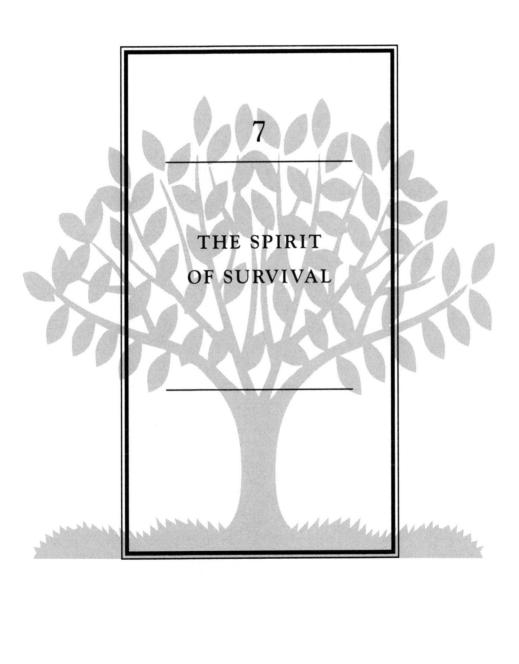

7

THE SPIRIT
OF SURVIVAL

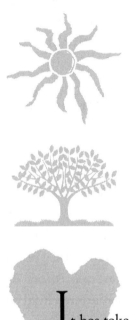

It has taken us a long time to begin shifting our focus away from why people die to understanding why people live. Despite mounting evidence that there is something about exceptional patients that makes them survivors, the medical profession still tends to focus on why people die, rather than on why some people beat the odds and live. We found that to be very much the case with Alex. No one studied Alex to determine why he made it. But, I guarantee you that if he had not, a necropsy would have been performed, and his blood, his kidneys, his brain cells, his spinal fluid, and probably a lot more of him would have been studied for years to come.

As we watched Alex waste away before us, we wanted to know *how to make him live*, not how the disease was killing him. We wanted to know ways in which we could help him, ways in which we could instill in him the will to live. Focusing exclusively on those who die—asking questions like, "What else could we have done?" "What did we do wrong?" and "What could we have done better?" assumes that medical treatment is primarily devoted to explaining the cause of death. Our experiences with Alex have convinced us that it is not all that simple. Miracles do happen, I'm sure of that. But beating the odds, I believe, involves more than a miracle.

Tapping into Your Child's Spirit

All the time Alex was in the coma from the bacterial infection, we talked to him as much as possible. I asked every approachable doctor and nurse—probably at least a dozen of them—whether they thought Alex knew we were there and whether he could hear our voice. Every single one said yes. I asked them if our presence would make a difference to his recovery. They all answered yes without hesitating. But I still wondered if they were just telling me what they thought I wanted to hear, so I did some reading. I found out that patients under general anesthesia do indeed hear what is being said. The content of what they hear, either positive or negative, clearly affects their recovery time. I read account after account of how patients in comas or under anesthesia were helped by the presence of loved ones and caring doctors. I found it so amazing. "Why doesn't everyone know this?" I wondered. It made me want to walk through the crowded parents' waiting room and tell everyone, "Get up, don't sit here. Go in and see your child. Sit with him, talk to him, hold his hand." But, I didn't. They would have thought I was losing it. *Instead, I am writing this so that all parents who go through an experience similar to ours will believe in their own abilities to help their child heal from within.*

When Tom and I were together at Alex's side, we'd talk to him and to each other, but we would never discuss our doubts about his ability to recover. We wanted Alex to hear our voices and to know that we were there for him. Sometimes when I was alone, I talked out loud to him. I'd tell him what happened that day. I'd tell him about the construction site we could see from our sixteenth-floor hotel room. I'd describe the cranes, the excavators, and the army of dump trucks carrying the dirt away like ants. Other times I talked to him about his illness and what was happening to him, hoping for a sign, any sign, that he was still in the body lying there before me.

Over time, I found it increasingly hard to talk for hours on end with no response, but I couldn't escape the feeling that he needed for me to be there—to talk to him, to give him something to look forward to. I began sitting next to his bed, holding his hand and reading him the poetry of Robert Frost. Robert Frost, Alex, and I had something in common—we loved covered bridges, birch trees, and everything about Vermont. My love for his poetry went way back, as the first poem in grade school I ever had to memorize was by Robert Frost. So I began by reading one of my favorite poems, "Birches."

> . . . I'd like to think some boy's been swinging them.
> But swinging doesn't bend them down to stay

I paused and wondered, then hoped and prayed that Alex would get out of there intact so that he, too, could someday swing on trees and ride them to the ground. I thought about how my sister, Lynn, and I used to climb up to the top of the great hickory trees in our front yard on windy days. The "King" and "Queen" trees, we called them. I always shinnied up the trunk of the King tree, and Lynn took the Queen tree. We'd yell across to each other, competing with the wind. Up in the sky, clinging to the pliant hardwood tree as it whipped back and forth, leaves rattling all around me, made me feel like I was on top of the world. "Why, Alex," I asked, "are you being robbed of this experience?"

It's hard to describe, but I think Alex and I clicked that day with the poetry. I don't believe he understood what I was saying. I'm not sure the words had any meaning for him. Even though he was in a coma, I sensed he knew I was there. I was moved by the poetry, and I was moved by the fact that Alex was fighting so hard to stay alive. We were stuck in a medical nightmare together, but at that moment, we might as well have been out in the woods bouncing on fallen birch trees. I think Alex knew it. There was a feeling around him and his bed, like a premonition or an eerie sensation of warmth and belonging. It lasted for only a minute or two, until a resident walked by and said, "Boy, I wish someone would read Robert Frost to me." But, from that day on, I didn't need to ask any questions or read any more about whether our presence made a difference. I *knew* it did. I knew we were as important to Alex's recovery as the ventilator breathing life into him.

Love, Stress, and Sleeveless T-Shirts

Many people believe that the primary ingredient to healing and recovery is unconditional love—unbridled, unrestricted, unqualified love with no strings attached. Is it unconditional love that separates the survivors from those who die? I think as parents we all try to provide unconditional love, but I'm not totally sure it's achievable. Being honest, it is very hard to say I love my child all the time with no restrictions. Do I love him when he's thrashing and moaning uncontrollably and my nerves have been shot for the last two hours? Do I love him when he's destructive and tears his brother's wooden airplane into fifteen pieces? Do I love him when he floods the entire bathroom floor on purpose? No, I don't love him at those times. But I do always try to love him for what he is, and I do try to understand his perspective and why he does some of the things he does.

It taught me a lot about unconditional love when Alex's bowel died from the bacterial infection and a colostomy was performed. Probably one of the reasons he lived was that he did have a colostomy. In the early days of his illness, the *E. coli* injected a neurotoxin in his system that caused him to bleed uncontrollably through his ostomy site. As they kept pouring more and more blood, plasma, and platelets into Alex to keep his blood pressure up, the ostomy site effectively flushed the neurotoxins out of his system. So I should be thankful that he had a colostomy, right? In fact, I hated it. I hated changing the bags. I hated the toxic gas that puffed out of the little charcoal vent. I hated cleaning up the aftermath when he did a belly-flopper on the slide and split it open. I hated paying nearly seven dollars a day for supplies because our HMO would not pay for it (insurance companies pay for them to cut a hole in your stomach, but I suppose they expect you to go to Grand Union and buy Ziploc bags to catch the excrement).

I tried to be cool and casual about it, but I hated it. Alex didn't fight it. I'm not even sure he was fazed by it. He named it his "pop-pop bag" because I would always say, "One pop, two pop," when I snapped the bag on the wafer glued to his stomach. I couldn't help myself for being nervous for him. While we were in the hospital, the ostomy didn't bother me; it was just another medical device like a feeding tube, an IV, or a catheter. But with the prospect of going home, it aroused all kinds of anxieties. How would I keep him from trying to pull it off? How would we explain it to other preschoolers? (Marty and I had already read *Chris Has an Ostomy* dozens of times, so I knew this was going to be no easy task.) How would we bathe him or take him swimming? "I'll deal with it," I thought. "I have to."

The first thing I tried to do was find him some sleeveless undershirts to tuck into his underpants to secure and cover the bag. It was no simple task in September in New England, and it became an obsession with me. I went into store after store in Lebanon, New Hampshire, near the hospital, and all I could find were girls'

T-shirts with lace straps and tiny pink rosebuds in the center. The last stop I made was in K-Mart. I went to the boys' underwear department. No luck. I went to the girls' underwear department, hoping I might find some neutral-looking undershirt. No luck. I was so frustrated that I stood there and exclaimed out loud, "Tell me, why is it that they only make these sleeveless T-shirts for girls?"

A saleslady overheard me and came over. I repeated the question and then proceeded to unload the whole story on her. Alex was in the hospital, he had contracted the "Jack in the Box" illness and almost died, had a colostomy—the entire story of our lives for the last two months. By the end, I was in tears and she nearly was, too.

"Deary," she said, taking me by the shoulder. "I think we have something that can help you." She led me over to the super-super-discount rack strategically positioned near the front of the store—all items $1—and said, "I think we have some little boy's tank tops left over from last summer." Like finding the missing ingredient for a soufflé, like making a computer program work after hours of debugging, I had finally found what I was looking for—blue ones, orange ones, black and white ones—it was a sight to behold.

Unconditional Love Sounds Good

When we were finally released from Dartmouth-Hitchcock Medical Center after the bacterial infection, we were determined to restore Alex's daily routine to as normal as possible. He was still sporting a feeding tube in his nose, through which we had to infuse high-calorie liquid nutritional supplements several times a day with an oversize plastic syringe. His foot was still bandaged from plastic surgery required to repair an area of skin on his ankle damaged by the bacteria. And, of course, he had his ostomy, now nicely covered and secured by a bright turquoise undershirt. Within two weeks of being home, we had ditched the feeding tube with the blessing of his pediatrician because he had begun to eat by himself again. His plastic surgery site was healed and no longer needed to be covered, although it still looked like he had been attacked by a mad wolf.

To restore his strength, we started taking him swimming every afternoon at the local health club. He had been going swimming there nearly every day before he got sick. When the staff of Timber Creek Health Club heard of his illness, they sent him cards and generously extended his membership for another three months. When we got home, he couldn't wait to get into the water again. We had discussed swimming with the ostomy nurse before leaving the hospital, and she had ordered some miniature, flesh-colored ostomy bags designed for swimming. I took him and Marty over to the health club for the first time since we had been home. Alex was a bit unsteady but went right over to the side, jumped in, and began swimming with the aid of his water wings. It was wonderful to see him swimming once again and to see his self-confidence returning. Afterward in the women's locker room, we ran into a mother and her four-year-old daughter changing to go swimming. "Mommy, what is that thing on his belly?" she said, staring and pointing at Alex.

I thought about ignoring the comment. Alex appeared to have ignored it, but the girl asked it again. I looked over at her mother in the mirror and decided to bail her out this time. I explained to the little girl how Alex had been sick, how he had had an operation on his belly, and how he had to wear this little bag instead of going to the potty like her. She squirmed a little during my explanation, and I could tell she couldn't wait to get out of the locker room. The next time we went to the pool, and every time thereafter, I put a black tank top on Alex, which he wore in the water— "My swimming shirt," he dubbed it. I found it really hard dealing with all of this. I couldn't help it, but it changed not only the way I viewed Alex, but how I had to manage his physical and social needs on a day-to-day basis. When he was well enough to start preschool for the first time that fall, I went in and instructed the teachers on how to care for his ostomy. I gave them a copy of *Chris*

Has an Ostomy to read if the other kids had any questions, but I had the feeling that most of them read it for themselves.

It disturbed me a bit that Alex's ostomy bothered me but not him. As much as I tried to say to myself, "This is a part of my child now, and I should love him for it," I couldn't. Unconditional love, I thought, was a nice ten-dollar word but, like self-actualization, was something you aspired to but rarely achieved. Despite all of my intellectualizing, I still felt like I was a failure as a mother. I wonder in retrospect if I would have felt the way I did had I not known his ostomy was reversible.

Over time, Alex became so comfortable with his ostomy that he began to parade proudly around the women's locker room at the health club showing it to everyone. If I was really lucky, there would be a group of senior citizens at the club that day who understood it, like the silver-haired lady who said, "Oh, isn't that nice. My husband, Marv, has one, too." We tried to share Alex's enthusiasm for his "pop-pop" with him, but it was not easy. Six months later, when we told him he was going for an operation to reattach his colon, he cried and cried. "Don't take my pop-pop, don't take my pop-pop," he said over and over. Tom tried to tell Alex he would be glad it was gone when he was older, but the logic of the argument was lost on four-year-old ears.

It was with truly mixed feelings that we took him to Dartmouth-Hitchcock Medical Center for the reattachment surgery. It was the first time he had ever gone to a hospital healthy. Plus, we clearly wanted his ostomy reversed and he didn't. All of us—Tom, Marty, and I—walked with him down to the operating room. I remember his frail little arms and pointed elbows sticking out of the pale blue hospital gown. I remember him clutching the strawberry-scented anesthesia mask he had chosen. Despite all that he had been through, I had never seen him look so frightened. I held him as they gave him the initial sedation, hugged him with all my might, and handed him to Tom to walk him into the operating room. Tom came back crying. So was I.

ON BEING AN EXCEPTIONAL CHILD

So why did Alex live? What is it about him that makes him a survivor? Why do other children die, even though their parents give them the same level of love and encouragement we gave Alex? You can look at Alex and tell he is an exceptional patient. One glance at him in his swimming shorts and it is obvious he's been through a lot. There is the long incision line that trickles down his middle, the puckered skin and jagged scar on his belly where his ostomy site once was, the white polka-dotted scars that mark the sites of chest tubes, central lines, and catheters, and the large crinkly scar on his ankle. But you don't really even need these landmarks to tell he is an exceptional patient. It is in his very being.

Alex is a kid who could easily be humorless, given all that he has gone through, but he finds humor all around him and his laughter is infectious. He likes to read books in the backseat on long car trips. On one trip, we bought him a new *Clifford* book, *Clifford and the Grouchy Neighbors*. Paging through the book, he came upon a drawing of Clifford the dog sucking up a nasty cat with a water pipe like a vacuum cleaner. He let out such a howl, followed by five minutes of uncontrollable giggling, that Tom nearly drove off the road. And, he's the best kid in the world to take to the zoo. Once at the polar bear exhibit at the New York Central Park Zoo, he started laughing at the polar bear doing flips in the water. Soon we were surrounded by a crowd of waist-high kids, all giggling with him and jockeying to get a better view. All the activity made him laugh even harder. He talked about that polar bear for days.

Alex lived, I think, because he has a survivor's personality, because he has parents and family that care about him deeply, and because he has a lot to live for. Life entertains him so. He can spend an entire day, if we let him, following a salamander over rocks, through the grass, and into crevices. He can lie on the kitchen floor with his dog, Curly, telling him stories for hours on end. When Curly dozes off, he taps him, commands him to wake up, and picks up the story where he left off. Sometimes I wonder if Alex really understands how short his life could have been . . . or may yet be. It seems to me to be a pretty complicated thought for a six-year-old. It's really hard to tell if he enjoys life so much because he almost lost it or whether he's alive today because life is just too much fun to give up.

Becoming an Exceptional Child

When I think about the traits of adults that make them survivors of life-threatening illnesses, I think of self-love, a sense of self-esteem, and the ability to face one's fears. One professional describes the survivor's personality as one of a "happy child"—curious, imaginative, self-absorbed in activities, with the ability to find humor in life. I don't know about your child, but it sure sounds a lot like Alex. Young children like Alex don't bring the baggage to their illnesses that many adults do. He has not experienced the disappointment of love not returned or a career gone awry. He's not afraid to cry. He's not afraid to share his feelings if he can express them and to admit his fears—I hear about them every day. In some ways, it is these qualities in children that make their illnesses or injuries seem so tragic. But it is these qualities that also give children an incredible advantage over adults when it comes to healing.

Can you as a parent make your child an exceptional child? I think so. I think every child is an exceptional child, but it is only a few, like Alex, who are truly tested. Allow your child to be a child—it will help tremendously. Be there and truly listen to what your child is saying and feeling. You can be upbeat, supportive, loving, and hopeful. You can be solemn and playful, serious and silly. These are behaviors that will let the goodness of your child come out. With it will come the tenacity to beat the odds, if indeed they can be beaten. Will it always work? No, but I wish it did. Someday I hope we will better understand why people live, not just why people die—and why some kids, like Alex, live against the odds. Until then, we have to accept the fact that some things are just not meant to be. As a parent, you never go wrong by trying to make the most of the time you are given with your child.

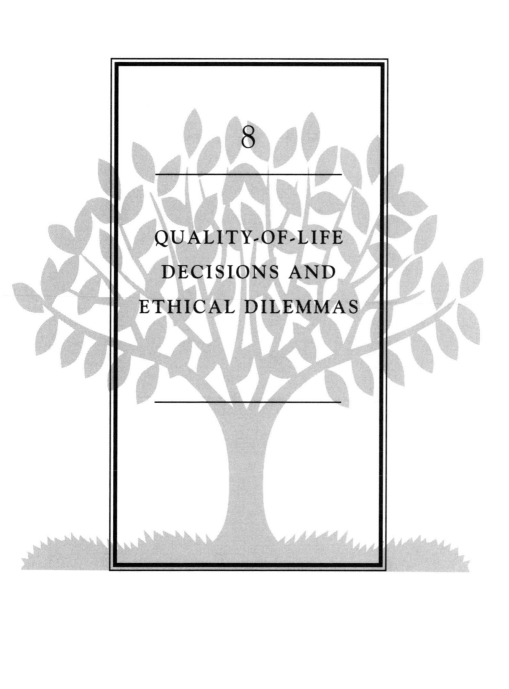

8

QUALITY-OF-LIFE
DECISIONS AND
ETHICAL DILEMMAS

Life-and-death choices are not straightforward—they try the souls of those affected. I don't like to admit it, but at one point in Alex's illness, Tom and I entered the gray, murky world of the threshold between life and death, living and being. It was our third morning in the ICU at Children's Hospital in Boston, and it will always remain the most memorable day of my life.

At 5:00 A.M. the phone rang in the communal parents' room, where we were sleeping. We knew it was for us even before a man wrapped in a sheet yelled, "Cain." The night before, Alex's blood pressure had begun to fall. We had gone to bed, unable to bear sitting helplessly at a distance from his bed while a battery of nurses and doctors worked on him.

"I knew it," whispered Tom as he stumbled in his underwear to answer the phone. The desk nurse simply said, "Please come to the ICU *now*." We kept bumping into each other, frantically trying to thread our jeans on in the dark in the tiny space between our cots. I was shaking so much that the simple act of putting on my socks was daunting. We raced into the ICU, where it seemed like every available adult was crowded around Alex. The room was dimly lit for nighttime conditions, but the lights surrounding Alex's bed space were blazing.

"I guess this is it," Tom said quietly to me.

I nodded my head, for no words would come out—only tears. The most senior resident took us aside and explained that there was no more they could do for Alex. He told us that he had called the attending physician, who was on his way in, and he would soon be there to talk with us. Tom and I needed to be alone together, but there was nowhere nearby to go. LouAnn, the nurse in charge, led us into a nurse's office overlooking the ICU. She brought us steaming-hot cups of tea and a big box of tissues. We had got to know her well over the past few days and had heard all about her son Tony, who was around the same age as Alex. We had traded stories and laughed with her, but now we were crying together. I'm not sure who cried more, Tom or me. Tom and I had known each other over twenty years, yet this was the darkest moment we had ever shared together. Nothing else, not even the untimely death of his sister over fifteen years before, had come close.

DNRs and Four-Leaf Clovers

When the attending physician arrived, he was joined by Jed, the blood banker. By that time, LouAnn had moved us to a conference room outside the ICU for more privacy. Tom and I were sitting together in shock, in the dark, when the physicians entered. They reviewed Alex's condition and sincerely apologized for not being able to do more. The big question we faced was, what do we do next, if anything? We reiterated the position that we had held all along—that we wanted everything possible done for Alex as long as there was any hope he would survive neurologically intact.

I remember Jed responding, "Don't worry, you're talking to nihilists."

I guess in that regard we were lucky. Too often, we had read nightmarish stories of people with no more than brain stem level of functioning being kept alive because someone thought it was "right." They didn't consider the patient's life or the lives or feelings of the family. Karen Quinlan was the most celebrated case, and Tom and I had agreed that the very last thing we wanted was a repeat of that. Alex was out there lying unconscious on a hospital bed. A respirator was breathing for him. Chemicals, now at their maximum levels, were keeping his heart pumping. His liver and kidneys were in failure. Ten different pumps were pouring medication into him, and he was bleeding uncontrollably from his ostomy site. How could we ever assess whether the Alex we knew was still inside that body?

The attending physician asked us if we wanted to issue a DNR order—"It means 'Do not resuscitate,'" he said. I closed my eyes and shuddered, wondering how it had come to this. Tom and I had talked theoretically about the issue of discontinuing support so many times since the night we first arrived in Boston. Now it was real—too real. Neither one of us wanted to make a decision. The night we arrived, one of the residents had told us, "Alex will tell us which way he is going to go." She didn't really have any medical basis to make that statement, but it sounded good and comforting. I clung on to that statement like a life raft.

"Alex is going to make the decision, not us," I had told Tom over and over. He had tried to reason with me. He had tried to tell me that it doesn't always work that way, but I didn't want to hear it. Just as Tom had warned me, we were now being asked to make a decision.

"I'm afraid I will make the wrong decision," I cried.

"Me, too," Tom sobbed.

Back and forth we went, spilling our most deep-seated thoughts. The two physicians listened and answered our questions. I had sounded so confident and brave the first night when we were asked, "So, how much do you want done for your son?" Now I was a mess. I just couldn't decide whether it was time to let go. Obviously neither could Tom. Were we being selfish using up more blood products and resources on Alex when there might be other kids needing them more? Sensing our inner conflict and indecision, Jed spoke: "Listen," he said, "we just started a new bag of platelets. Let's finish the infusion and see where we are."

We all agreed that approach made sense. Jed and the attending physician said a few comforting parting words and then left Tom and me alone in that dark conference room to confront our demons. It was 6:00 A.M. I reached over, picked up the phone, and called my family to tell them not to bring Marty to Boston that day because Alex probably wasn't going to make it. My sister, Lynn, later told me that my family spent the day at our house in solitude, unable to escape the ghost of Alex's impending death. As a child, Lynn was an ace at finding four-leaf clovers. She has always had that ability to gaze at a scene and instantly spot something out of order. She said she went out that morning for a walk by herself and collected as many four-leaf clovers as she could find—it was a bouquetful and all she could think to do to help.

The Miracle

Tom and I sat in the conference room and waited for the final word, but in our minds Alex was gone. We kept asking ourselves over and over how this could have happened, how were we going to go on living without him? His illness over the past week had already made such a hole in our lives. We had only seen Marty once during that week, but it was so hard to be around him because he was an unforgettable reminder of what we had been as a family. I thought about a remark a fellow parent had made to me on the sidewalk just the day before. He was pushing a stroller down the street toward the hospital—it was a triple stroller, with a bouncy eleven-month-old child in the front and an identical one asleep in the back. The middle seat was empty, for the third of the triplets was in the ICU with Alex, recovering from surgery for the removal of a cancerous brain tumor. We stopped on the sidewalk briefly to ask each other how it was going. We were both sporting hospital beepers and dark circles etched under our eyes, so clearly all was not well. In parting, he sort of blurted out, "We used to have a perfectly matched set," and looking joylessly at the empty seat, added, "No matter how this turns out, it will never be the same again."

That was now how I felt. We had been the typical two-parent–two-child family—the kids never outnumbered us, although it sometimes seemed that way when they acted like wild animals. And we never outnumbered them. Marty and Tom, both blonds, looked alike, had the same mannerisms, and had always gravitated toward each other. Alex, with his dark brown hair, brown eyes, and squared-off jaw, looked more like me. He and I were soul mates in the same way that Tom and Marty were. We, too, were a matched set and I didn't think I was ever going to recover from the loss of Alex.

It takes a plump bag of ruby-red blood about thirty minutes to trickle into veins the size of Alex's. That was the window we were looking at, but Tom and I had lost all sense of time. As much as we had thought it through and talked about the likelihood of Alex's death, we couldn't believe it was really happening. It left both of us in a dissociative state—we felt like we were simultaneously the actors and the audience in a play, watching an unreal drama in which we were the players unfold in front of us. When there was a knock on the door, I stiffened, realizing that the time had come.

In walked Jed and the attending physician. If I hadn't been so distraught and felt so disconnected, I probably would have noticed that they entered more with a jaunt than the sluggishness of defeat. They sat down and told us that the most amazing thing had happened. Just as the last of the blood was trickling into Alex, he suddenly stopped bleeding and his blood pressure stabilized. Yes, they were nihilists—they had said that right up front—but we all sat there for a moment wondering whether we had experienced a miracle.

POSTSCRIPT

Tom and I have never got over how close we came to losing Alex and to making the wrong decision. We learned a lot from that experience. More than anything, we learned that it is truly impossible to tell anyone else what to do in a similar situation. But I think there are things about our experience that are worth noting. *Nobody made any decisions for us.* Luckily they didn't try, for we wouldn't have let them. *No one pressured us or chided us for our indecision.* Rather, Jed and the attending physician listened, without trying to interject their opinions or lead us one way or another. To them, for their compassion, their intellect, and their patience, we will forever be grateful. I only hope that other parents who find themselves in a situation like ours will be as lucky as we were, to be able to deal with outstanding people like them. We took all of the time we needed to think through what was happening—to be clear in our minds that we understood and were at peace with what we were doing.

We didn't involve anyone else in our thinking, neither our families nor our friends. It was a private decision that we had to make on our own, and our thoughts will forever be held in the four walls of that conference room. What anyone else thought didn't matter, for we were the ones who were going to have to live with the consequences. Probably the only other person who had a right to be in on the decision was Marty, but it wasn't a decision in which to involve a child.

In the end, I was right, or at least partially right. Alex made the decision. He or something far greater than he or all of us chose for him to live.

In the Soul of the Decision

We later discovered that Alex had nearly died three times before that early morning in Boston, when he once again hovered between life and death. When he first arrived in Brattleboro's emergency room, they couldn't get a blood pressure reading—it was so low that the digital readout was blank. During emergency surgery at Dartmouth, his blood pressure once again dropped to the floor. Unable to continue with the surgery, the surgeon stapled him together with a few large wing clips for the night and resumed surgery the next day. We also know that he barely lived through the trip from Dartmouth to Boston, although no one was ever specific about exactly what happened. It must have been pretty bad for the attending physician to greet us with the statement, "How much do you want done for your son?"

Tom and I have often talked about how different it would have been if Alex had died in Brattleboro's emergency room or the following day during surgery at Dartmouth. We would have had an entirely different perspective on doctors and hospitals. They would have been technicians and institutions to us, not healers and places of hope. We never would have felt we had any control over what was happening, and that would always have left us lonely, dissatisfied, and wondering. We never would have understood the anguish involved in thinking about making life-and-death choices. It is something you can never understand until it happens to you. Hopefully, it never will. In reality, Alex wasn't snatched from us like a bolt of lightning—it was a slow, agonizing, soul-searching journey through hope and despair, culminating in a miraculous recovery.

We had the time to think things over, and in our own way, experienced the grief that comes with the loss of a child. We progressed through many of the stages associated with grief: shock, anger, guilt, despair, questioning, healing, and renewal. As it turned out, Alex did not die, but some part of us did. Somewhere between Brattleboro, Dartmouth, and Boston, we left parts of the "old" us on the cold cement of the ambulance dock, on the hard benches outside the ICU, and in the fog hanging over Boston on the night of Alex's arrival. But, just as I believe in life after death, I believe that Tom and I were changed for the good and, in turn, have changed others around us. I think we appreciate life and what we have more. I think we understand ourselves better, even if at times we look into our souls and are disappointed with what we see. More than anything, I think we are more sensitive to the ethical issues involved in medicine. Life-and-death choices are not straightforward. Indeed, they are not.

At Peace with Yourself

At the times when you must make difficult decisions, I think it's very important to believe in yourself and to trust your own instincts about your child. Whether you are making a life-and-death choice, a decision for your child to have elective surgery, or a decision to continue or discontinue a treatment, you need to feel that it is right for you as well as your child. What has always worked for us has been to first make sure we were as informed as we could possibly be. We talk with as many physicians as possible to get different opinions. We talk to nurses, therapists, and anyone else who works closely with our child. Then, when we've collected and digested all that information, we talk with each other and go with what we know best—our intuition.

Sometimes you are called upon to make a decision concerning

your own child's well-being that does not necessarily involve a life-and-death matter. Even in those circumstances, it pays to listen to your intuition. Alex had his first seizure just three weeks before Marty was born. I was a very stressed second-time mother, to put it mildly. I had been hospitalized with breakthrough bleeding during week 30 of my pregnancy with Marty, and my obstetrician had decided to deliver Marty three weeks early, particularly in light of Alex's medical problems. Luckily, Marty's birth turned out to be uneventful. Tom had the baby-sitter stay at home with Alex, and Tom and I were able to experience a birth the way we thought it was supposed to be—magical and wondrous with no hint of medical problems. Things went so smoothly that Marty and I went home after two days, C-section and all.

The one problem I had was that Marty would not nurse. Maybe it was because I was under so much stress, or maybe it was an early indication of his obstinate personality, but he refused to cooperate. "Don't give him a bottle," the nurses on the maternity ward said. They sent the hospital's lactation expert in to see me, which wasn't much help. "He'll nurse when he's ready to," she said. Once at home, I voiced my concern to my pediatrician. "Don't give him a bottle," he said. But Marty wouldn't nurse and it was making me even more nervous because he seemed like he was starving. I used a breast pump to express what little milk I had and tried to drip it into his mouth. On the fourth day, he began to look emaciated and was terribly cranky. I did what I thought was right. I whipped out a bottle, mixed up a formula and breast milk cocktail, and gave it to him. He sucked it down without stopping.

I thought about all of the stress I had in my life at the time, and this constant hassling with breast-feeding was creating more stress than I could handle. But I felt so guilty for giving in—all the books, the experts, everyone was touting the wonders of breast milk. A La Leche League bumper sticker I saw even read, AFFORDABLE HEALTH CARE BEGINS WITH BREAST-FEEDING. They made me feel like I was ruining my child's life for years to come by giving him that evil baby equivalent of junk food—a bottle of formula. But, regardless of how bad I felt, I knew I was doing the right thing for Marty. His weight since birth had fallen more than the expected few ounces—it was more like a pound. At around five pounds and twenty-one inches in length, he had a face that looked skull-like and he felt more like one of those stringy sock-monkey toys than a newborn.

The next day, my pediatrician called to see how Marty was doing. He asked how the breast-feeding was going and I told him how I had given up and was feeding Marty bottles of expressed breast milk mixed with formula. There was silence on the other end of the line, and I could just imagine him going, "Tsk, tsk." He reiterated the importance of breast milk to early health and nutrition, while I silently fumed. I couldn't believe that this guy, of all people, the person who had treated Alex three weeks earlier, who had seen how sick Alex had been and the stress we were under, could be so unsympathetic as to make me feel guilty. It wasn't his child whose life had been threatened by a seizure and was still staggering around, overloaded with antiseizure medication. It wasn't his child whose cheeks were sunken and wouldn't nurse. In fact, he didn't even have any kids of his own. "Someday," I thought, "he'll understand," and I left it at that.

Last year, I happened to read an article on the front page of *The Wall Street Journal*, of all places, headlined, "Dying for Milk." It told the story of a mother who tried to breast-feed her newborn and was having problems. Everyone, from nurses on the maternity ward to her pediatrician to a breast-feeding consultant, advised her to keep trying and not to resort to formula. When her son was six days old, he suffered dehydration-induced brain damage—permanent brain damage. "I can't stop asking myself," the mother said, " 'Why didn't you ignore all of the experts and give him a bottle?' "

Although this is not the only case like this, it is an extreme one that illustrates the importance of going with your own instincts when it concerns the health of your child. Unfortunately, first-time mothers are far from confident and often feel vulnerable. I know I was when Alex was born. I was admonished in my home by a baby nurse for buying regular cotton balls rather than sterile ones. When I asked her what difference it made when she poured them into an open container on the changing table anyway, unsterilizing them in the process, she "tsked" at me. So I, *not she,* hobbled out to the neighborhood pharmacy and bought sterile cotton balls. (But I did fire her after the second day of a week-long engagement.)

When Marty wouldn't nurse, I figured it was probably my fault. When I looked at his sunken eyes and hollow cheeks on the morning of his fourth day, something in me snapped and said, "He comes first." You know what? It made me feel a lot better, and there was no question that if he could have talked, he would have said something like, "Thank you, Mommy. Whatever took you so long?" For the next twenty-four hours, it seemed like he ate constantly. He became more active and it was once again possible to look at him without feeling pain. I learned to deal with the judgment of my pediatrician. I learned to ignore the hostile glances when I fed him a bottle in public in our politically correct neighborhood. I went with my instinct, and I know it was the right thing for *both* of us.

Organ Donation and Other Thoughts

From the time Alex arrived at Children's Hospital until the morning when he came so close to dying, we really had no idea where he was going. He'd have periods of instability when his blood pressure would drop precipitously. Then following a transfusion, he would seem to coast for a while, not getting any better, but not getting any worse. It was during this time period that we had a long honest talk one afternoon with a resident named John. John took a personal interest in Alex's case. He followed every detail and became a tremendous source of knowledge and support for us. He would always make a point to visit Alex's bedside a number of times during the day. He never seemed hurried or impatient and would tirelessly answer the zillions of questions I had. I guess it was because of his easygoing manner that I blurted out the question to him one day, "If Alex dies, can we donate his organs to another child?"

It was something that I had been thinking about a lot. I had looked around the ICU and seen so many children in critical condition. I was desperate to find something positive in Alex's illness. I told him I realized Alex's liver and kidneys weren't of much use, since they were currently in failure. But we had been told that he had a very strong heart and we wondered how we might go about donating that to another child. He thought a minute and then shook his head. No, he thought, no one would dare take the risk of transferring what was left of the *E. coli* bacteria to a heart-transplant candidate. It was likely the neurotoxin was still in his system, he said, plus Alex had received blood from over fifty different donors by now, which would make it risky as well. Suddenly the disease made me furious and I started ranting and raving about how evil a bug this was. It was bad enough that it was sucking the life out of my child, but the fact that it was trashing his body forever seemed so unjust. Not only were we not going to get our son back, but it was going to be a terminal illness in the worst sort of way.

John listened sympathetically to my rage and frustration and then added that maybe Alex's eyes could be donated. I don't know whether he said it just to make me feel better or whether it really was a possibility. Thankfully, we didn't have to find out. But John did thank us for being so unselfish and thinking about organ donation. He told us that not many parents in similar circumstances are willing to consider it. He wished that more parents felt the way we did.

When I thought about that scene after it was apparent that Alex was going to recover, I realized that I wasn't being unselfish at all. I had come to grips with the fact that I might lose Alex, but I thought that maybe a part of him—a physical part—could go on living in another child. Yes, a potential recipient, a child whose life depends on a donated organ, might view it as an unselfish thought. But for me it would have been the beginning of the healing process, knowing that my child had died but had given another life. I recently read about a man who willed his body to a medical school. It was Dartmouth. He said he always wanted to go to Dartmouth and he did, as a cadaver. I guess that was a possibility, too, should Alex have died. But, I can't help wonder what a first-year anatomy student would have thought of a body swollen out of recognition and so utterly trashed by a little bug that lives innocuously in the environment around us.

Tom and I know if we or our children are ever in a position where it makes sense to donate our organs to someone else, we will be the first people to step forward and offer. We've seen too many children dying in ICUs, hoping that an essential organ will become available before it's too late. We've been inspired by the young children we encountered in the dialysis unit who had the courage to keep fighting until a kidney became available. This experience made us realize how lucky we were that Alex's kidneys restarted. Otherwise, he, too, would be tethered to a children's hospital, waiting for a kidney along with the others.

What Are We Saving?

Perhaps Tom and I viewed Alex's illness and hospital stay with more awareness of medical ethics than others, but I don't think so. We just articulated more openly what a lot of people think and feel. I remember the testy discussion we had with an attending physician over why a CAT scan couldn't be done on Alex's brain while he was still on a respirator. I remember my frustration at the catch-22 situation: "We can't tell you whether the bacteria has destroyed his brain until we save him." It wasn't until I pointed out the dilemma the medical staff was creating for us that they agreed to do the CAT scan anyway. Would they have insisted on "saving" him first before assessing what they were saving had we not made such a stink?

Alex's primary day nurse, Mareaid, busied herself organizing Alex's many tubes and leads while she listened silently to our conversation with the attending physician. When he got up and left at the end of our discussion, Mareaid spoke out assertively in her Irish accent, "You know, I think you two are doing the right thing. I admire you for that. Too often in here [the ICU] everyone gets carried away with saving a life without really thinking about what we are doing."

It was quite a statement. But I was glad to hear her say it, even though I found her admission troubling. It made us realize how important it was to think through the medical issues. It also made us glad that we had spoken up, although we recognize that in other situations it might be more prudent to keep your feelings to yourself.

The subject matter of this chapter is not easy to discuss. On many levels, it has been the most painful aspect of Alex's illness for me to write about. But ethical issues are something that need to be discussed. Dealing with life-and-death issues for a child is perhaps the most agonizing of all. You have to look at the potentially long life ahead of him or her and your entire family. We wanted the child back that we brought into the hospital—we didn't want the cocoon of our child. But that was our choice. *Only you know what is right for you.*

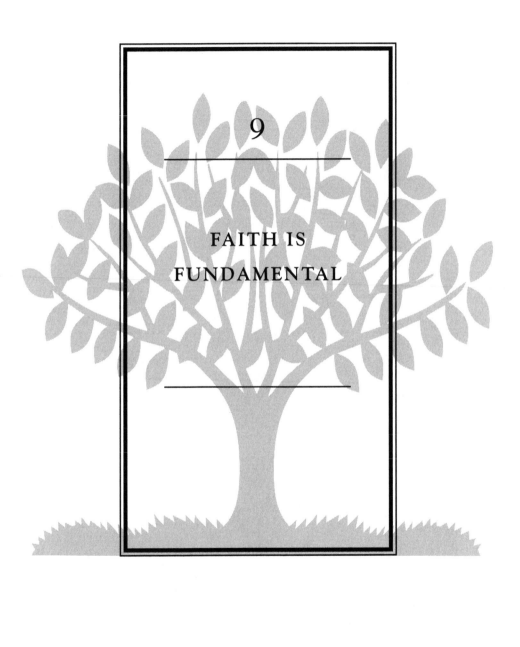

9

FAITH IS
FUNDAMENTAL

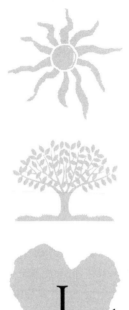

In my heart I know there was something more powerful at work in Alex's illness than medicine, more profound than unconditional love, and more enigmatic than the human mind. I'll be the first to admit that I simply don't understand it. I do think, however, I know what carried us through the ordeal. We got a tremendous amount of support from our family and friends, as well as total strangers. But beneath it all, it was faith and the steadfast conviction that we could make a difference that were our greatest sources of support. To me, these are the real ingredients of healing.

Going through all the motions—sitting with your child, holding, touching, talking to your child, and even getting the best medical help available—is not enough. You must have faith and truly believe you can make a difference. How you derive that faith, be it from your religion, your family, your friends, or medical expertise, is not what is important. It is the positive energy that your faith creates. I can't tell you the number of parents and medical personnel who actually came out and said they were inspired by our courage to continue despite the odds. They used such words as "strength," "aura," and "togetherness" to describe what I believe is the positive energy we helped bring to Alex's healing process. This positive energy can't help but inspire others, including your child, to reach just a little higher.

Keeping the Faith

It is hard for me to describe what it really felt like to know that my child might die any minute. I had never felt so alone in my whole life, maybe because it was the first time my faith had ever been tested. I remember sitting on the hard window bench outside the pediatric ICU at Dartmouth during the first day of Alex's illness with the *E. coli* infection. I was huddled up uncomfortably with Tom sitting next to me. Tears flowed continuously from my eyes. One moment I was sitting there in shock and the next thing I knew, a toothless old woman with stringy brown hair and a musty smell had thrust her face into mine. "It's all in God's hands, it's all in God's hands," she chanted. Then she stepped back as suddenly as she appeared and was gone. At first I thought she was an apparition, my delirious mind playing tricks on me. What was she? Who was she? Was she some bizarre harbinger of the truth? She turned out to be the grandmother of another child in the ICU, and her intrusion into my personal space and our life made me furious.

The incident instantly transformed me from a limp, pitiful parent to an angry, defiant activist. "What an idiot! What an *incredibly* stupid thing to say," I said.

"I'd like to strangle her," Tom added.

At that moment, I knew I had faith, but I also knew that the faith was not blind. "It is not God's will that Alex die," I thought. "Why would God want a young, happy child to die? If it is all in God's hands, why are all of these medical people working night and day trying to save him? Why even bother with medicine? To believe it is all in God's hands is to give up faith. And who are God's hands, anyway? Aren't they the loving hands of everyone who has touched him during the last twenty-four hours?" In retrospect, I should have answered the woman with another spiritual homily: "No, you're wrong. 'God helps those who help themselves,'" for that statement is to me the essence of what it means to heal . . . or to be healed.

Alex has one of the most peaceful fighting spirits I have ever known. Never before have I witnessed a person so serene yet so determined to get the most out of life. I think it was largely in his spirit that we found faith—the strength to keep fighting for him, the faith that we were doing the right thing, and the belief that we as a team could make a difference. Through his illness, our spirit and his became one, dedicated to the grueling process of survival, recovery, and healing.

SUPPORT FROM OUR FAMILIES

I don't think the faith to help your child heal comes naturally for everyone. It certainly didn't for me. I think it is something we acquire through our life experiences. It comes from simultaneously being a parent and a child, from learning through our personal victories and defeats, and from struggling to make our hopes become realities. The support of other loved ones can steer you through difficult times, through periods when you doubt your ability to add positive energy to your child's healing process. For many of us, one of our most important sources of support is our families.

I remember how angry we were with an extended family of grandmothers, aunts, uncles, and cousins who raucously partied in the parents' waiting room at Children's Hospital while their child lay in the ICU with Alex. They came in as a crowd one Sunday afternoon, toting a cooler of drinks and bags and bags of potato chips. We wanted to shoo them out of there. We wanted to scream at them to be quiet. We wanted to get up and turn off the deafening football game they were watching on the TV. But we didn't do any of those things. We just retreated into a conference room and waited until we could get back into the ICU to sit with Alex. We realized we didn't have a right to be angry, for support for that family clearly was different than for us. We wanted to be alone—to reflect on what was happening in solitude. The other family was dealing with their grief in their own way—almost as a family wake.

We know we would not have made it through the first week of Alex's illness had not my mother and sister been there to take care of Marty. But over time, it was very difficult for us being in Boston, an unfamiliar city, far away from family and friends. Not being able to see Alex and not being able to be with us made it difficult for our families to truly understand what was happening. At the time, we had parents and siblings living all over the country—in Houston; Los Angeles; Charleston, South Carolina; Chicago; Sperryville, Virginia; and Ithaca, New York. As immediate family, they wanted to help us out, to be there for us, and to be updated the moment Alex's condition changed. But having family at a distance wasn't very satisfactory. When we talked on the phone with them, they couldn't see our red-rimmed eyes, our hands shaking from exhaustion, or the despair draped over our entire beings. They couldn't reach out and hold us.

As the days progressed and grew into weeks, it became harder to talk with our families every night on the phone. There was nowhere to talk privately, for we had abandoned what little privacy we had by choosing to stay at Alex's bedside during the day and to sleep in the hospital at night. We felt we had a responsibility to keep our families informed, but it became increasingly difficult to repeat the same information over and over. It drained what little energy we had, and we couldn't afford that. Everyone had well-meaning advice for us, but we didn't need advice. We needed to be held. We needed for someone to watch over and take care of us in the same way that we were taking care of Alex. To maintain our sanity, we fell into a routine where we called one spokesperson for each side of the family every night. That family member, in turn, called and relayed information to everyone else. Even with this system, our phone bill at the end of the first month was a staggering $300.

Using family spokespeople to relay information about Alex reduced a lot of our stress. For days we had been dogged by well-meaning phone calls that always came at the wrong moment. We were so distraught that we couldn't help but interpret innocent questions as if our or the medical staff's judgment were being second-guessed. Often, we'd hang up the phone feeling worn out and frustrated. One day sitting at Alex's bedside, Tom was visited by a priest sent to see him by a family member trying to help. It threw Tom badly, and instead of adding positive energy to the situation, it made Tom feel as if the priest had come to begin the burial process. Until we got through the "touch-and-go" portion of Alex's illness, what worked for us was to keep our extended family at a distance. We know that won't be true for everyone, but I think it's a good idea early on to ask yourself which of your communications with family members are helping the situation and which are creating additional stress.

FRIENDS IN NEED ARE FRIENDS INDEED

Our families, our friends, and the entire congregation of our church kept up the vigil, saying prayers for us, sending gifts and touching notes, and keeping our home back in Vermont from reverting to nature. That support allowed us to focus all of our energies on Alex's healing and recovery. But over time, we found ourselves increasingly alienated from the outside world: our families, our friends, and our acquaintances with perfectly healthy children. How could they begin to understand what we were going through? Inside the hospital, we found a different kind of family—parents of other hospitalized children, the medical staff who cared so fervently about Alex's well-being, and total strangers who reached out to us in simple ways that said, "I care." Those who had been through it themselves and those who read the daily anguish on our faces like a book provided the level of compassion and support we so desperately needed.

During breaks or whenever we weren't allowed in the ICU, we would sit in the parents' waiting room. When other parents would ask us about our son, we would describe how he had contracted the "Jack in the Box" illness. The illness at the time was still pretty much thought to be a West Coast phenomenon related to eating undercooked hamburger. Thus, other parents would shudder and pull their children closer to them when they heard that Alex's was the only case of *E. coli* 0157:H7 in Vermont that summer, and that he had contracted it from an unknown source. They always wanted to know exactly what the bacteria did to him, and we took to describing him as a "train wreck," explaining how all of his vital organs had failed. One day, after Alex had been moved out of the ICU onto the medical floor, Marty met another preschooler in the playroom and they became friends. When I asked the boy if he had a brother or sister in the hospital, he told me that his older brother was there. I asked him what was wrong with his brother and he told me that he had gone on a Boy Scout hike and had been hit by a train. I never described Alex as a "train wreck" again.

I don't think any of us in the waiting room realized how important it was for us to talk about our children's illnesses until we shared the information with one another. We talked a common language—hi-fi respirators, CAT scans, chest PT, and the like. We shared common concerns and fears: Would our children live? How much longer could we take living in the hospital? Were we going to run out of money? Would the ordeal ever end? We talked openly about the deaths in the ICU. Practically never a day went by that we weren't herded out of the ICU in a panic as the staff attended to a medical crisis or another child's death. We couldn't help but compare our child's condition with that of the one who had just died. We couldn't help but wonder if our turn were next.

Despite all the frank conversation and the gloominess of our situations, the parents' waiting room was usually a place of hope and healing. It was a place where we confronted the reality of our children's conditions. It was a place where we listened to others and others listened to us. It was a place where we traded medical knowledge and tips on the ins and outs of dealing with certain doctors and nurses. We inspired other parents to keep going, and they in turn inspired us to forge on. We visited some of the bed spaces of the families we got to know well, and they visited Alex's. Other parents found beauty in Alex's swollen, distended, and maimed body—it was the beauty of hope, determination, and life itself. We also found beauty in the shaved heads, miles of sutures, and connections to complicated machinery of other children—it was the beauty of courage, of medicine at its best, and of the will to live.

The parents of other hospitalized children helped us feel more at ease. We didn't have to make any excuses for Alex's condition or Alex's behavior. During his recovery, we didn't have to explain why he was drooling or why he couldn't pick his head up or why he acted more like a newborn than a four-year-old. We didn't have to worry about the reaction of other children or the impolite stares of strangers. In the hospital we lived in a bubble, a distorted bubble, where the labels "normal" and "abnormal" lost all of their meaning. The minute we encountered even the most well-meaning friends or family, we felt the need to make excuses, to qualify everything. More than anything, we found the outside world dwelled on the future, as in "Is he going to recover fully?" or "Is he going to experience developmental setbacks?" Answering these questions, for which we still don't know the answers, created an incredible amount of stress for us. It was no wonder that we gravitated toward other parents of hospitalized children for our day-to-day support. Like us, they had learned not to dwell on the future. Like us, they had learned to live one joyous day at a time.

Much later, when we discovered that Alex's bout with the *E. coli* bug was going to have long-term implications in the form of a life-threatening seizure disorder, the first person I wanted to call was Laura. Laura was the mother of Zach, a six-year-old who had been battling viral encephalitis for the past two years. We met Laura and her husband, Roger, during our stay in the ICU at Children's Hospital. For a while, Alex and Zach were two of the most hopeless cases in the ICU. Both of them lay in comas for weeks on end: Zach's disease had veered out of control into the world of one continuous seizure, and Alex's body was under siege from a tiny little bug intent on killing him. We spent a lot of time with Roger and Laura, mostly waiting, worrying, talking, listening, and instilling courage in each other. I knew Laura and Roger would understand what we were going through in a way that no one else would. To this day, despite the fact that we live very different lives in different states, we take the time to keep in touch with each other, to say we care.

Out of the hospital, I once tried replicating the experience of sharing feelings and concerns with other parents by attending an emotional support group. It surprised me greatly to find that I didn't feel much comfort in belonging to a group where we simply vented problems and issues. It wasn't that I was uncomfortable discussing my feelings, but rather that I'd grown too impatient to just talk about them. Alex's illness has brought out the activist in me: Today, I'd much rather be trying to solve problems than talking about them. I want to find ways to help us cope with Alex's illness. I want to find ways to prevent what happened to us from happening to others. I won't stop until I have educated parents, hospitals, entire communities, and political leaders, for I believe that helping a child to heal from within extends far beyond the bond between a parent and a child. But, just because an emotional support group was not good for me, it doesn't mean it's not good for others. I think local groups have a tremendous amount of support to offer, and I encourage other parents to at least give them a try.

Medical Personnel and Other Healers

For us, one of the most surprising sources of support was the medical staff and hospital employees. Somehow, we had an image of detached medical personnel—nurses and doctors who didn't get personally involved in their patients' cases. But our notions were far from reality. Jennifer, the nurse who washed, blow-dried, and coiffed Alex's hair when it wasn't clear he was going to live until the morning, was so supportive of us and so protective of Alex that she might as well have been a family member. Jennifer was the first person in the hospital who suggested that it might do both Alex and me good for me to hold Alex in my lap. When she first asked me if I wanted to hold him, I looked at her in disbelief and said, "Excuse me?" for I did not think that I had heard her right. I gestured at all the medical equipment he was connected to, the spaghetti wires pasted all over his body, the bilious tubes draining out of every orifice, and the miles of intravenous tubing.

"Not a problem," she said. "We'll just take it slowly and gently." Then she busied herself organizing all the wires and tubes. When she was ready, she sat me down in a chair next to his bed and carefully hoisted his warm, puffy, and toneless body into my lap. It didn't look, smell, or feel like Alex, but it felt wonderful to cradle him once again.

"That's the way it ought to be," said Jennifer, looking down at us. The tenderness in her voice made me realize that it felt as good for Jennifer to see Alex lying in my lap as it did for me.

And then there was the cashier in the cafeteria at Dartmouth whom we got to know. She wasn't a nurse, a doctor, or a chaplain, but she was very much a healer. The first time we encountered her, she asked the obligatory question, "Are you employees?" for employees received a substantial discount on their meals.

"No," we answered, "we have a very sick four-year-old boy upstairs in the ICU."

She read the suffering in our faces, winked, and gave us the discount anyway. The next day, when there was no line, she asked us what was wrong with Alex and we told her the whole story. Every day thereafter she always gave us the employee discount and asked how the "little guy" was doing. Sometimes she would reach inside her pocket for a quarter and buy Marty a chocolate chip cookie if we would let her. The day Alex recovered enough to visit the cafeteria in a wheelchair, she stood up in awe when she saw him coming. Teary-eyed, she patted his shoulder and told him to keep on fighting.

We never learned the cashier's name and she never learned ours. She will always be "the cashier lady," but someone we will never forget. She wasn't the only hospital employee who went out of his or her way to help us. It amazed us how much the nonmedical employees seemed to care. There was the chubby-faced janitor who would collect Mylar balloons left by former patients and bring them to Alex and Marty. And there was the "tray lady" who always left Alex's tray with the message, "May Jesus be with you." We found that emotional support was all around us and that healers and healing could take many forms.

Hospital Staff Support

Hospitals, of course, also have on their staff a number of traditional sources of support: the social workers, the child life specialists, and the chaplains. These are the hospital staff members paid to provide families like ours with any of the support services they need. All the social workers we encountered were invaluable sources of information. Think of a social worker as someone who can help manage your life inside the hospital: They can tell you where to stay, how to access sources of financial support, how to contact national support organizations for various illnesses, how to get around on public transportation, and lots of other tidbits of information you need to know to survive your child's hospitalization. We ended up using the social workers a lot—for simple things, like borrowing a stroller for Marty, and for more complicated tasks, like helping us negotiate the maze of forms necessary to qualify for meal, housing, and parking subsidies. If you are also dealing with Medicaid support or Supplemental Social Security payments, social workers are the people who can help you through the daunting amount of paperwork involved in accessing these programs.

When your child is in a hospital with child life specialists on the staff, you're lucky, for these individuals helped us tremendously in finding ways to entertain Marty and to stimulate and entertain Alex as he recovered. Child life specialists play many different roles, depending on the hospital. Some manage the process of educating and preparing children for their hospital stay, some oversee hospital playrooms and activity programs, some coordinate school-oriented tutorial programs for long-term patients, some help siblings cope, and some do a little of everything.

Marty still wears the Boston Red Sox baseball cap ("my Boston hat") that Suzanne, a child life specialist at Children's Hospital, gave him. He was down in the dumps one day, and she gave it to him to cheer him up. Now, it's one of his most prized possessions. Carolyn, the sole child life specialist at Dartmouth, works with the entire family, not just the patient. For us, she took the concept of family-centered support one step further—to the four-legged member of our family. During one long hospitalization, Carolyn took Alex's dog, Curly, home with her and kept him for several weeks until Alex was released. She knew we had enough worries to deal with, without having to worry about who was taking care of our dog.

Most medical facilities have at least one chaplain on their staff. The chaplain's role is to provide spiritual support for patients and their families. I don't think Alex has ever been hospitalized for more than several days when a chaplain has not stopped by to see us. Once during one of Alex's longer stays at Dartmouth, Mark, a particularly persistent chaplain-in-training, kept reappearing at Alex's room every day.

Mark had a perpetually boyish face and a soothing, whisperlike voice. He was so low-key that he practically glided into Alex's room unnoticed. I guess it was obvious that we were under a lot of stress and that Alex was not doing well. Mark decided it was his mission to reach out to us. He was the first chaplain we ever encountered who neither tried to impose his beliefs on us nor simply retreated when it was obvious that the visit was causing us discomfort. The first time he arrived, I was "talked-out" and exhausted, so I mechanically answered his questions, studiously avoiding any deeper discussion. He sensed I did not want to talk, but he continued to reappear every day and just sit in Alex's room for ten or fifteen minutes, bathing the room with his spiritual presence. I didn't know what to do with him, but I wasn't quite sure that I wanted him to leave. One day, he picked up a book and started reading to Alex to give me a break. That brightened Alex's spirits, and Alex began to look forward to Mark's daily visits. Oddly enough, so did I. Mark and I both realized that we didn't have to talk to connect with each other. Over time, his presence alone had a noticeably calming influence on both Alex and me.

SUPPORT IS ALL AROUND
(AND WITHIN) YOU

It amazes me when I think about how little Tom and I really knew about ourselves until Alex's illness. Our children have always meant a lot to us, but we didn't know how much they meant until we nearly lost Alex. We discovered faith in ourselves and each other that had lain dormant for years. We learned how important our families are to us, and how hard it is to live far away from them. Our lives were touched by so many supportive people—family, friends, acquaintances, and medical personnel—but we discovered it was hard work channeling all of the support into positive energy directed at Alex's healing. Initially, Tom and I naively thought that together we could handle Alex's illness on our own. We learned how much better it was for him and for us to share some of that responsibility. We learned that in helping others, we helped ourselves—that healing goes both ways.

I had always thought angels were white-robed, heavenly winged creatures with golden ringlets of hair and cherubic faces. They're not. The real angels are middle-aged cashiers wearing black hair nets; sun-tanned nurses with bouncy blond ponytails; bearded ambulance drivers with kind hands; and all the other people like them who breathed life into Alex and gave us the hope and the courage to sustain it.

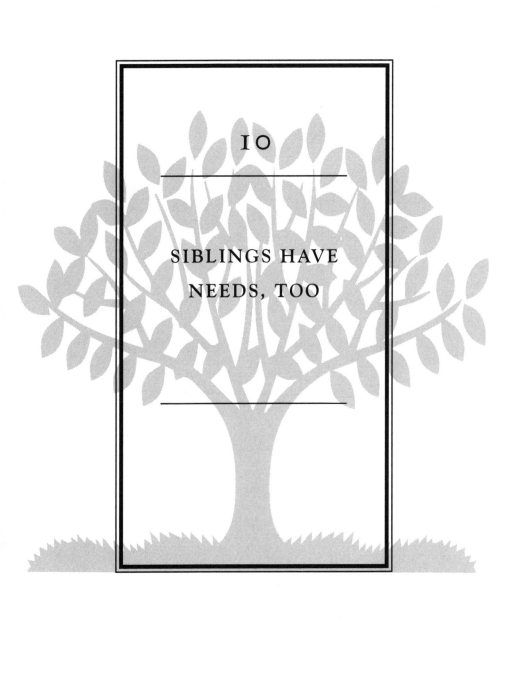

10

SIBLINGS HAVE
NEEDS, TOO

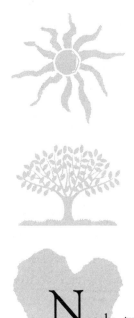

Nearly two years have passed since Alex contracted the *E. coli* infection. He has finally recovered from the immediate effects of the illness, but I'm not sure Marty ever will. The events of the morning the ambulance roared out of our driveway with Alex have changed Marty forever. I remember tearfully leaving Marty sobbing in my mother's arms, not realizing at the time that Alex was dying and never imagining I wouldn't see Marty again for days. I often wonder what I would have said to Marty, who was two and a half at the time, if I had had any idea of what we were about to go through.

During the peak of the crisis, we found it very hard to balance our need to be at Alex's side with Marty's need to be with us as a family and understand what was happening. In retrospect, I don't think we were as understanding as we might have been with Marty, but we did what we had to do. During the first week of Alex's illness, we barely spoke to Marty, and pretty much left it up to my family to explain to him what was going on. We've always believed in telling our children nothing but the truth, but I didn't really want him to know that his brother was dying. We kept Marty away from the hospital for two reasons: so that we could make difficult decisions without any distractions and so that he wouldn't see Alex. If he had seen Alex, who with his fluid-filled body and misshapen face looked more like a manatee than a child, he would have been terrified for the rest of his life. I know, because every time I visualize Alex at that stage of his illness, it makes me shudder.

When my family brought Marty to Boston for a short visit, we didn't want any of them to see Alex—we preferred that their last memories of Alex not be of some distorted-looking monster. Instead, we met my family in the outdoor garden at the hospital. It was a day more suited to a summertime picnic than grieving in a hospital garden ablaze with flowers. When Marty came running over, I picked him up, but it was hard to hold him. I loved him dearly, I had missed him so much over the past week, but at that moment, the child I really wanted to hold was Alex. I held Marty's sweet-smelling, squirmy body close to mine, and it made me miss Alex even more. I imagined how Alex would have oohed at the flowers and how he would have danced about the garden like a marionette. I couldn't help myself. All I wanted was to hear Alex's bubbly laughter and to hold him just one more time.

I remember Tom sitting on a bench between my mother and my sister. He might as well have been just another statue in the garden. He smiled weakly when Marty bounced excitedly in his lap and told him that Aunt Lynn had given him *sprinkles* on his ice-cream cone. Neither of us tried to talk with Marty about what was happening, for Marty appeared content just seeing us and exploring the garden paths. When the visit was over, we watched them drive away. I wasn't sad, I was numb. Tom and I talked about the visit as we walked back to the ICU. Tom told me how hard he found it to be around Marty—Marty reminded him of how incomplete our family would feel without Alex. His idea of family would always be "four," yet there would only be three of us. We both felt depressed and guilty and wondered whether Marty had picked up on our real feelings.

"Dr. Marty Party"

Nearly a week went by before we decided that Marty should come to Boston and stay with us—we felt it was important for our family to get back together again and deal together with Alex's illness. As inconvenient as it was to have Marty with us (we slept together on a tiny, one-person cot in the parents' room and Tom and I constantly had to keep an eye on him), he brought with him the cheery exuberance of a young, healthy child. The day he arrived, he started asking questions and never stopped. Some were purely informational like, "What's that?" "What's that for?" And some were much tougher: "Is Alex going to die?" "Will I get the same germs as Alex?" It was a little scary to see the amount of knowledge he amassed. Before long, he started accosting strangers in the elevator and trying to explain dialysis to them. One day, I happened to overhear him explaining how a breast pump worked to one of Alex's residents: "You see, the milk goes in here and goes round and round and Parmesan cheese comes out here." The day Alex was taken off the respirator for the first time, the whole hospital knew; Marty told them all.

It wasn't long before the entire medical staff in the ICU was charmed by Marty. Amidst the bleak atmosphere of the ICU, he made troubled people laugh with his buoyancy. He wore the stethoscope from the doctor's kit we'd bought him around his neck like all the residents and carried his black doctor's bag everywhere. Betsy, the resident who had received the lecture on Parmesan cheese, nicknamed him "Dr. Marty Party," and it stuck. Everywhere we went in the hospital, people knew him and called him by his nickname. We were glad Marty seemed to be adapting to Alex's illness so well—it was one less stress we had to deal with. As long as Alex was comatose and unresponsive, Marty thought he was the center of the universe and was charming and agreeable. But as Alex began to recover and started demanding more of our attention, we began to see a few cracks in Marty's facade. Marty had dealt outwardly with the stress of Alex's illness by becoming an entertainer. In return, he was lavished with the attention he craved.

As Alex grew more demanding of us, so did Marty. I'd be sitting reading a story and Marty would start with a long string of demands: "I'm hungry, I'm tired, I have to pee, I'm thirsty, I want to go to the playroom, I want to go for a walk." Tom and I took turns taking Marty out for the day to museums, parks, and playgrounds, but we still felt anger, hostility, and jealousy building in Marty. Periodically, Tom or I would take Marty home to Vermont, but he seemed moody and unsettled there as well.

What Is Normal, Anyway?

When we finally returned to Vermont at the end of Alex's illness, we were glad to be home and have things back to normal. But the problem was, things were no longer really normal. Alex had been a healthy, happy child and had come back weakened and insecure, with enough battle scars to win a medal. Marty got his first "big boy" haircut during that time, and along with the long blond wisps of hair, he lost his easygoing exuberance. He was now moody, demanding, and unusually competitive. On top of everything else, Alex's medical problems proved to be far from over. For the better part of the next year, he was in and out of the hospital, and it seemed like some calamity was always waiting for us on the other side of the door.

Marty became harder and harder to handle. We had never really seen much in the way of temper tantrums from him before, but even the most minor frustration like, "Marty, I'm sorry, but we are out of yogurt," would send him into a rage. When we tried to talk to him about why he was so angry, we discovered that he had no idea. The first thing we did was discuss in depth what had happened during Alex's illness and why Alex was still sick. In the hospital, Marty had acquired all of the vocabulary and learned to converse about Alex's illness, but outside the hospital it was obvious he still really didn't understand it. I think he expected the illness to go away when we left the hospital, and when it didn't, he was angry.

We acknowledged Marty's anger by letting him know it was okay to be angry and that we were sometimes angry, too. We explained Alex's illness in concrete terms he could understand. Not surprisingly, we discovered that Marty still felt responsible for Alex's sickness. We assured him that Alex's illness had nothing to do with him. We also talked with professionals, who told us that it was typical for a child of his age to equate love with the amount of time a parent spends with a child. We had been spending an inordinate amount of time managing Alex's illness, and Marty clearly felt less loved. Now that we were home, we knew if we didn't correct this imbalance, our problems with Marty were only going to get worse.

During the year after Alex's illness we truly lost sight of what was normal. We kept Alex in our bed at nighttime because we were so afraid he was going to have a seizure in his sleep. This troubled Marty greatly and made him feel left out. As a young child, Marty had often awakened us singing in his crib, happy and full of energy. Now he was waking up angry and disagreeable every morning. We did the only thing we could think of: One of us began sleeping with Marty in his bed and the other with Alex in our bed.

Instead of rolling over and kissing each other good night, Tom and I would pause in the doorway between the two rooms, kiss each other good night, and climb into bed with one of the kids. If someone had made a sitcom of our lives at that time, no one would have believed it. It took us nearly a year and a half to convince

Marty that it was okay to sleep alone and that we were not having a nocturnal party every night that he was missing. Over time, we praised Marty for being a "big boy" and let him know that big boys preferred sleeping alone. Now Marty finally accepts the fact that Alex slept with us because he had to, and Marty has returned to his old roosterlike self in the morning.

IT WAS MY FAULT

About six months after Alex's illness, we had several days of springlike weather, a February thaw, despite the fact that the ground was still blanketed with four feet of snow. I ambitiously shoveled for hours until our back deck was clear enough for the kids to play outdoors. Tom took the kids outside to play, and Marty lugged his ride-on truck with him. Tom was standing by the railing not five feet from Alex, gazing into the woods when he heard Alex let out a dreadful scream. He looked over and saw Alex lying on his back with his leg tangled in the railing. Marty was sitting on his truck at Alex's feet looking down. Tom reached over and picked up Alex. When he did so, he realized that Alex's foot was pointing in a very odd position, and he was sure it was broken. Over Alex's piercing screams, Tom tried to ask Marty what had happened, but Marty wouldn't talk. Tom took Alex inside, stretched him out on the bed, and called me.

After a trip to the emergency room, where Alex received a full-length cast on his leg for a broken tibia, Marty finally admitted that he had backed Alex into the railing with his ride-on truck. Marty has never really said whether it was an accident or not—he won't say, so it was probably a little of both. For a time after that incident, Marty's anger seemed to turn to guilt. The event confirmed some of Marty's worst fears—that he was partly to blame for Alex's illness. It didn't help matters that Alex began having big seizures. Ambulances appeared routinely at our house, Alex was hospitalized for days at a time, and doctor's office visits became as routine as going to the grocery store. In all honesty, we were quite angry with Marty for what had happened, but we gave him the benefit of the doubt and treated the incident as an accident. But from that point on, we were more careful to watch Marty's interactions with Alex for two reasons: We wanted to make sure that Marty was not intentionally trying to hurt Alex, and we were afraid that Marty could accidentally injure Alex in the course of playing, since Alex was so frail.

Dr. Spock Is Not Much Help

Dr. Spock wasn't able to help us much in managing Marty's reaction to Alex's illness, nor were the social workers and professionals we spoke to on a casual basis. I've discovered they don't write child-care books for exceptional cases like ours, and I've never yet found a professional with a quick fix. On our own, we realized that Alex's illness was not just Marty's problem but our entire family's as well. We should have been joyous that Alex had beaten the odds and lived, but all we really felt was stressed and exhausted. When people heard our story, they would inevitably tell us how lucky we were. As many times as I heard it, as often as I came to expect it, I never could help myself from looking at them incredulously and saying, "Lucky?" The people I found particularly difficult to deal with were the parents who had lost a child. They never failed to tell us how lucky we were, and on many levels I knew they were right. But what they and many others just didn't understand was that we, too, had lost a child—the child we had hoped and expected Alex would be.

Our free time following Alex's hospitalization was nonexistent, and our relationship with each other suffered as a result. Our entire lives were centered on Alex's medical needs and Marty's emotional adjustment. It didn't matter what we talked about—our families, something we had read, our careers, the future, or even the weather—the vanishing point of our conversation always seemed to be Alex. I can't tell you the number of nights we put the kids to bed and asked ourselves why we ever had them in the first place. We would try to discuss how to deal with the next calamity or outburst, often with one of us falling asleep in mid-sentence on the couch. Both of us admitted we fantasized about getting in the car and driving off, never to return, but we both knew we could never do anything like that to each other or our kids.

Despite the stress, we tried to be as supportive of each other as possible. We had nursed Alex through a near-death experience and were doing our best to help Marty through his difficult adjustment to Alex's illness. It didn't leave much energy for each other, so we tried to spend as much time with each other as possible, to the exclusion of outside activities and friends. Tom and I dealt with Alex's illness very differently. I needed to talk about it and I needed to be hopeful and optimistic. Tom humored me and let me talk and cry for hours on end when I needed to. Tom, on the other hand, needed to brood on his own, and although he was not overtly pessimistic, he was always much more guarded than I about getting his hopes up. I responded to his needs by giving him space. We both shouldered the burden of Alex's illness and Marty's reaction equally, but we did it in our own ways.

What's a Typical Sibling Response?

Alex's illness gave us very few choices. With a critically ill child, the concept of being a "superparent"—a parent who works, makes sure his or her children are healthy and happy, keeps a spotlessly clean house, and has a hot, well-balanced meal on the table every evening—went right out the window, along with everything else associated with traditional families. Just getting through a day at a time seemed like an insurmountable task. It was a very difficult time for all of us, and it was Marty's emotional adjustment in the end that suffered.

Marty's behavior convinced us that there is no typical sibling response to another sibling's illness. In discussing our situation with other parents, the only thing we found in common was that all of us were having problems. Some siblings were angry, some felt neglected or jealous, some were becoming unusually aggressive, and some were withdrawn, irritable, or detached. It didn't seem to make a difference how old or what sex the child was; each one was reacting in his or her own personal way. The fact that Alex's illness was not really visible to Marty (except Alex's ostomy, which Marty dismissed with, "I hate that smelly thing—it makes my nose hurt") made it all the more difficult for him to understand why Alex needed additional attention.

In talking with Marty, we realized that behind his angry, temperamental behavior was intense fear. He wasn't afraid to witness one of Alex's grand mal seizures. Nor was he bothered by blood, needles, or surgical wounds. What frightened him was the fear of the unknown. Despite his young age, he had a need to see, hear, and understand every detail of Alex's medical condition. As much as we tried to explain things and as much as he personally witnessed, it never seemed to be enough. Sometimes it almost seemed as if he were cross-examining us. It took a great deal of patience and repetitive explanations to make Marty feel he was informed. If he didn't understand something fully, he made it up. He was (and still is) the kind of kid who could invent scenarios in his mind that were far more frightening than reality itself.

"Dr. Marty Party" Becomes "Arty Marty"

I'm not quite sure when Marty's interest in art began. I'd like to think it started when Alex was in the ICU at Boston and Marty turned out one "masterpiece" after another for Alex. Before we allowed Marty in to see Alex, we suggested to Marty that he draw some pictures as a way of getting him involved in Alex's healing process. We told Marty we would take his artwork into the ICU and hang it in Alex's bed space. When Alex came out of the coma, he would open his eyes and see Marty's pictures, and they would help him get well sooner. Marty decided that this was a fine thing to do and set to work with paper, crayons, scissors, and glue.

When we first allowed Marty into the ICU at Children's Hospital in Boston, his first remark was not about how horrible or strange his brother looked, but how interesting the ICU was and how pleased he was to see his artwork hanging around Alex's bed. It was several days later that Alex opened his eyes for the first time. I was sitting at Alex's bedside when his eyelids slowly parted and opened wide. I squeezed his hand and called out his name as he drifted in and out of consciousness. For days we had sat at his bedside, hoping and praying for just this moment. He finally came to, just long enough for me to get a tiny response out of him, and then he slipped back into unconsciousness. I was so emotional that I went running out of the ICU and burst into the waiting area to tell Tom, who was playing on the floor with Marty.

"Alex opened his eyes," I said loudly. "He wiggled his toes for me!" In the background, a talk show was blaring from the TV, but I distinctly remember seeing all the faces in the room riveted on our drama instead.

"Alex saw my picture! Alex saw my picture!" Marty said, hopping up from the floor. "Alex opened his eyes and saw my picture."

I don't think anything else in the world at that moment could have given Marty more satisfaction. By the time Marty was three and a half, he had gained a great deal of fine motor control and had begun drawing representational art. By his fourth birthday, Marty was drawing elaborate pictures of space scenes, complete with all of the planets, the sun, asteroids, spaceships, and aliens. Everyone began to notice Marty's artistic talent, but more important, Marty noticed that everyone noticed. Art became an obsession with Marty. To this day, the first thing Marty wants to do when he gets up in the morning is draw.

In Marty's mind, Alex has special needs, but he has a special talent. It seems like such a simple point—that Marty needed to feel special like Alex—but we managed to almost miss it. It's not that we didn't try to give Marty special attention, because we did. We would do little things with him only, like taking him swimming or taking him for pizza. We bought him little gifts whenever Alex was hospitalized and let him pick out the books in the library. But it never seemed to work, for he just responded by raising the ante. He begged for more attention and bigger and better gifts. What we didn't see at the time was that none of the things we were giving him made him feel special. The feeling of specialness had to come from inside Marty himself—it wasn't something that we could give him like a present. That was quite a realization for us. From then on, we tried to better understand Marty, the person, not Marty, the brother.

Understand Me for What I Am

Over time, it has taken us a lot of trial and error to figure out that we need to understand Marty on his own terms. We have learned that he can adapt to Alex's illness and our preoccupation with it without creating havoc in the family. But first, we had to listen hard to what his behavior was telling us—that he needs to be special, he needs to feel helpful, and he needs to understand every detail in order to feel in control.

When you are so focused on the needs of your ill or injured child, it is all too easy to tune out what your other children (or your spouse, for that matter) are trying to tell you. Marty's needs—to be special, to be helpful, to understand, and to feel in control—are universal needs for every child with an ill or injured sibling.

When it comes to managing sibling relationships in your own family, the best advice I can give you is to pay attention to these needs.

Alex's illness took our entire family by surprise and was far more traumatic for Marty than we ever imagined. It is unfortunate that Marty practically had to shout to be heard. It is not that we didn't recognize Marty was having problems. The temper tantrums, the nightmares that left him dripping in sweat, and the almost daily questions about death were clear warning signs, but we naively thought they would go away with time. They might have, had Marty not been reminded of the trauma again and again by Alex's continuing medical problems. In focusing all of our energy on Alex's recovery, we left Marty by the wayside. I think we realized at the time that the healing process transcends recovery and involves far more than the body and the mind of the injured. What we originally failed to recognize was the extent to which Marty was "injured" as well.

This is as much a story about Marty as it is about Alex. There is something about siblings, about brothers only eighteen months apart in age, that links the fortunes of one so closely with that of the other. It is a relationship of love and hate, worship and envy. I see the jumbled feelings come spilling out in Alex's and Marty's interactions nearly every day. It is not easy under normal circumstances to be the younger sibling. I know, for I was once the competitive younger sister living in the shadow of my sister, Lynn. The day Alex caught the deadly *E. coli* bug, Marty caught it, too, in another way. Alex's illness has changed the way Marty thinks about himself, but most of all, it has changed the relationship between him and his brother. Marty will always be the younger brother, but he will also be the healthier one. For that I'm sure he will feel fortunate, but will it ever be without the pain of guilt?

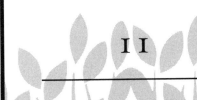

II

THE HIDDEN LIVES
OF CHILDREN
WITH MEDICAL
CONDITIONS

Alex's illness did not end with recovery from the bacterial infection; in some ways it just metamorphosed. During Alex's illness, we insisted that every neurological test be done, and little of any significance was found. It was, therefore, astonishing to us to find that the illness left Alex with a difficult-to-control, life-threatening seizure disorder. Maybe it was the acute swelling of his brain caused by the illness, or the prolonged periods of perilously low blood pressure, or the septic shock caused by the death of his bowel, or the reactivation of a seizure disorder diagnosed earlier in his life that lay dormant for nearly two years. We will probably never know the real cause. Of his current seizure disorder, his pediatrician says: "I have yet to encounter a child with more dramatically frightening seizures."

With every seizure, we confront the very real possibility that it may leave Alex permanently impaired, retarded, or even dead.

Many people ask us, "How do you deal with it?" Sometimes we're not sure how we do, but we know we neither are alone nor by any means have the worst situation. There is a whole group of us out there who have children with debilitating and life-threatening medical conditions. We live very different lives from families with healthy children, and we make whatever adjustments we have to in order to create a safe, warm, and livable environment. We also get used to functioning at a high level of stress. It is no wonder that the divorce rate for families of children with medical and physical impairments is astonishingly high.

When I think about the stress we live with on a day-to-day basis, it reminds me of an event that occurred during my first business interview many years ago. It was with a recruiter from Citibank, a huge barrel-chested man, dressed in an impeccably pressed navy business suit. His presence was so overpowering that he made the interview room seem claustrophobic. I was the third person on the sign-up sheet to meet with him. After the first person interviewed came staggering out of the room, word quickly spread that the recruiter was using a style known as a "stress" interview—a rapid-fire barrage of questions that left you gasping for breath. "What did he ask?" I asked my limp colleague. He told me the toughest question was, "Have you ever been in a situation where the contingencies changed overnight?" I mulled that over a bit and decided the recruiter wanted to know how we handled stress.

When it was my turn, I walked confidently into the room and was hit with a series of questions as soon as I sat down. Then came the question about changing contingencies. I paused for a moment, to let him think that I was giving it some thought, and then gave him my spontaneous-sounding but rehearsed answer. He stared directly into my eyes with a look of "This is war," and coldly said, "That's nice. Now tell me about another situation." I quickly made up some lame response. Needless to say, I didn't get the job.

It still makes me laugh when I think back about how I let that recruiter intimidate me. My life has changed so much since then that I often wish I could look him up and have him ask me the same question again. This time, I would answer him with another question: "Have I ever been in a situation where the contingencies *didn't* change overnight?" for this is what our life with Alex has become. That recruiter had no concept of what stress really is. I know business can be stressful. I once was a foreign exchange trader for all of six weeks when I made a $5 million mistake. That was stress all right, and it was a pivotal event in deciding that trading wasn't for me. But it was child's play compared with what Tom and I have experienced with Alex and what we continue to deal with on a day-to-day basis.

Life in the Control Tower

A more appropriate occupation to describe what it is like to raise a child with a life-threatening illness is that of an air-traffic controller. You must keep your eyes on your subject and never look away. You must constantly be vigilant, and you must never let your guard down, for lives depend upon you. Being an air-traffic controller is a stressful job with a high burnout rate for which the work conditions are monitored carefully. When an air-traffic controller reaches his or her limit for attentiveness, someone comes in and provides relief. But, this is where the jobs of parent and air-traffic controller differ. There is never anyone who can truly relieve the burden you carry as a parent.

When we have people over to our house for the first time, they come expecting to see our own little *Rescue 911* setup, but our situation is not that obvious. At first glance our house looks like anyone else's. The kids play in Alex's room, but no one notices that the bed often hasn't been slept in for a long time. If they look hard, they might notice that our children have more than the usual number of medicine-oriented books, or that our kids' favorite bathtub toys are oversize plastic syringes. They may stumble upon our stash of emergency medication in the butter holder of our refrigerator, but that's about all. Behind the facade of normality is what they don't see: the closet next to our bed full of emergency equipment, including oxygen tanks, a regulator, pediatric oxygen masks, tubing, an ambu bag (for manual resuscitation), syringes, vials, and a stethoscope. And they don't see the overnight bag always packed for a hospital stay and the list of emergency phone numbers taped prominently inside the closet door. On the surface, our life seems as normal as possible, and we work incredibly hard to make it that way.

It's difficult for other parents and friends to understand what we really go through. "He looks healthy and robust to me," they all say when they meet Alex for the first time. Few people notice the small insulated bag of medication we take everywhere, in much the same way a Secret Service agent trails the president with a hot-line phone. They register surprise when they ask us whether we've seen a new movie and we tell them that we haven't been out together alone in the past eighteen months. "You don't have a baby-sitter?" they ask. It's hard to make even the most compassionate person understand that we couldn't nor wouldn't ask a baby-sitter to be responsible for getting Alex to the hospital forty-five minutes away in a life-threatening situation.

It Changes the Way You Sleep

Sometimes we amaze ourselves at the accommodations we have made in our lives, all because of Alex's medical condition. We've changed the way we live, the way we work, the way we think, and for a while, we even changed the way we slept. At night, we used to take Marty to his room, tuck him in, and say good night. Then we'd take Alex to our room, which had by default become his room, too, and tuck him in. Later, when we went up to bed, we'd have to move Alex and all of the things he'd taken to bed with him over to his side of the bed with the railing. I always slept next to Alex, for I sleep lighter than Tom. I never went to sleep at night without first listening closely to make sure Alex was breathing and wondering if we would make it through the night. To this day, when Alex has a cold or a fever, we increase his antiseizure medication, and he sleeps with us. Every time he tosses, coughs, or turns in his sleep, I wonder if this is it. If I sound a little paranoid or overly cautious, I am. Four times now, I have been awakened by a seizure.

Alex used to fight us when we tried to put him to bed. "I want to sleep in *my* room," he said. "I want to sleep in my own bed with my own striped blanket." How do you tell a six-year-old that he can't sleep in his own bed because you are afraid he might die in his sleep? Once, we tried letting him sleep alone with a monitor. Then he caught a cold, and we put him back in our bed for a few nights. The second night, something about him woke me. I turned on the small flashlight I keep under my pillow and saw that he was swallowing repetitively and silently smacking his lips. Then, within seconds, his body convulsed and he went into a full-blown grand mal seizure that only medication could stop. So much for the monitor. It never would have picked up the sounds or behaviors that preceded the seizure, and he probably would have been gasping for breath before we heard it. By then, the seizure may well have been too severe to stop with just the emergency medication. And so, Alex sleeps with us if he is sick or if for any reason we suspect something may be wrong.

It Changes the Way You Work

Tom and I used to live in New York City, where the children were born. I worked for a major money-center bank and Tom for an investment firm. Our typical workday began with a ten-minute walk to the subway at 8:00 each morning and often ended long after darkness with a ride home in a "black car"—a corporate equivalent of a taxicab. And that was when one of us was not working all night on a transaction or traveling. At times, both Tom and I traveled nearly once a week. How could we have managed our jobs and Alex's medical condition? We couldn't have even if we wanted to. As progressive as corporate America would like to think it is with regard to the family, it has a long, long way to go. There is absolutely no way our employers would have accommodated our personal situation, and on some levels I can't blame them. I understand the difficulties associated with having an employee that you can't rely on at all times. If it came down to Alex's life or a multimillion dollar deal, no matter how important it was, Alex would always come first.

The way we make our livelihood now as writers allows us the flexibility to manage Alex's medical condition. When Alex must be away from home—in school, for example—one of us is always close by and available by phone in case of an emergency. In the afternoons after school, a baby-sitter watches the kids while we work upstairs in our offices, within earshot of any calamity. If necessary, we write at night and in the early hours of the morning. We always try to use our work time as efficiently as possible, for we never know when we will have to drop everything, sometimes for days at a time.

HAVING AN ASTERISK NEXT TO YOUR NAME

Inevitably, the unconventional lifestyle we live has led to some degree of social isolation. Although they don't really come out and say it, other parents seem to be a little afraid of dealing with Alex.

And while they are planning play dates and sleepovers for their kids, we are not. My friend Dotty, who has a child with developmental delays, deals with some of the same concerns. She describes the feeling as "having an asterisk next to your name." That's a fairly good description of what it feels like to raise a child with special needs in a small town. We realize that the day will come when we can no longer protect Alex, medically, socially, and otherwise. One day, we fully expect Alex to ask to go on an overnight camping trip with friends. We only hope by then that we have a better understanding of his illness and how to control it.

There are also those people who think because we work at home for ourselves we are retired. And there are those who look at our flexible work hours and the time we spend with our children and think we live a charmed life. If only they knew what it was really like. When we signed up for parenthood, I think we had a good idea of what we were getting into, but we never, ever imagined how tough it could be dealing with a child with a life-threatening condition. I also had the naive belief that "lightning never strikes the same place twice," and it is still hard for me to believe that Alex could have ended up with both a life-threatening seizure disorder and a deadly *E. coli* bacterial infection. Not only have we dealt with his long-term medical problems, but we have agonized through the ups and downs of a nearly fatal illness. Our life behind the scenes is about as charmed as a trip to the dentist. We do our best to ensure that we live as normal and as happy lives as possible.

It Means Always Being Prepared

Life with a child like Alex means always having to have a plan. During the last winter in our old house, for example, it snowed for several days, then rained, then froze, then rained, and froze some more. Our house at the top of a hill on a private dirt road was iced in, and it made us fairly nervous. On top of everything else, Alex had a bad cold and a sinus infection. "What if we had to get out of here?" I asked. Tom decided we should drive our four-wheel-drive vehicle down to the town road to check on the road conditions. He backed out onto the road and we slid the entire way down the hill until we crashed into a snowbank near the bottom. The hill was too icy to drive back up, so he parked it at the bottom. Clearly, the roads were not good. I then walked (or rather slid) the rest of the way out to the town road and found it had just been sanded. So we developed a plan. If Alex had a seizure, we would call the ambulance, administer his emergency medication, and place him in a flat-bottomed plastic sled and cover him with blankets. We would then pull him down the hill to the car and drive him out to the town road to meet the ambulance.

We have plans for the snow, the ice, and the mud, and we have plans for handling an emergency by ourselves or together. We've made sure every member of the rescue squad knows where we live, and we've been in the Brattleboro emergency room so often, they know exactly what to do when they hear Alex is on his way. We never go hiking, skiing, or canoeing without emergency medication and thinking through a plan for getting help. When we drive somewhere, we favor highly traveled or well-known routes, and on longer trips, we map out our journey ahead of time, taking into consideration the spacing of towns and hospitals along the way. Sometimes it seems like we have more plans than the military, but we have to—for Alex's safety and for our own peace of mind.

EVERY FAMILY'S SITUATION IS DIFFERENT

Some children have predictable life-threatening illnesses and others do not. Alex's illness falls into the latter category. Although he is taking maximum doses of antiseizure medications, they don't always control his seizures. We always have to guard against complacency, for it is often when we think things are getting more manageable that we are thrown off guard by a seizure. On the playground, we can never relax, for the simple act of falling and bumping his head can trigger a life-threatening seizure. And, we always must be on the lookout for the first signs of a cold, virus, or infection—more often than not, his seizures have been triggered by minor events like these. But we also have to recognize that Alex is an active six-year-old like any other. He can't live in a bubble, for there is more to life than just being. So what do we do? How does our family handle his situation?

We've found physicians we trust and who trust us. Between the combined efforts of our pediatrician and our neurologist, we keep close tabs on Alex's health, neurological development, and medication levels. We've learned to schedule blood tests around the workday of Michele, an empathetic lab technician who reads Alex's veins with the skill of a navigator. We never have to fight for medical attention—in an emergency, we get an instantaneous response, and even when he shows the slightest signs of getting sick, an appointment time is always made available. Our physicians trust us to administer huge doses of a powerful sedative in the event of a seizure and to regulate his daily medication up or down, depending on his health and behavior. We work as a team, always willing to try new approaches and never giving up on our quest to discover the underlying cause of his seizure disorder.

We've built up our own medical knowledge. Not long after Alex was born, we enrolled ourselves in a pediatric CPR course, a step that I recommend every parent take whether he or she has a child with an illness or not. We learned how to perform CPR effectively, but, more important, it gave us the confidence to manage an emergency situation. I can't tell you how many times we've had to rely on the knowledge we gained in that course to stabilize Alex's condition. We've read about seizure disorders and tried to relate our knowledge to Alex's specific condition. We've been trained by our neurologist to look for signs that precede seizures and for subtle behaviors manifested during seizures (e.g., was he looking to the left or right?), and we've learned the importance of timing in all of our actions. We've educated ourselves on the actions and interactions of various medications and the role of dietary factors in seizure management. We've been trained on the use of basic life-saving support equipment, including oxygen tanks, regulators, pediatric masks, and ambu bags. Out of necessity, we've become a self-taught First Response team, and I can say in all sincerity that Alex would not be alive today had we not.

We insist that everyone who deals with Alex is educated on his condition. We go to great lengths to ensure that school personnel, therapists, baby-sitters, friends, other parents, and backup physicians are apprised of his condition. Inevitably, we also have to provide a lot of support in the form of equipment and recommended actions to ensure these people are not afraid to work with him. The ability to recognize subtle changes in Alex's mood or behavior is paramount. Catching the beginning or warning signs of a seizure can make a tremendous difference in its likelihood and severity. Our educational plan has paid off. In five different instances, it was either someone working with him at preschool or a caregiver who detected the onset of seizure activity.

We actively work to reduce stress. We have one big enemy in our struggle to live our lives as normally as possible and that is the buildup of stress. We are both runners and have been for over fifteen years now. Exercise, we have found, is our best form of stress management—we do our best to pound our worries into the dirt and gravel of the roads that traverse the hills around our home. In running, we find not only the stress reduction that comes from physical activity, but the time to be alone, think alone, and enjoy the beauty and solitude of the spectacular place in which we live. Raising a child with a life-threatening medical condition doesn't give you much time to yourself, but one of the most important pieces of advice I can give to someone in a similar situation is, take care of yourself and make the most of the time you have.

Alex's life-threatening medical condition has changed our lives. There's no getting around the reality of it on a day-to-day basis. There are a lot of things we can't do that others do. We are often forced to make accommodations that others might find intolerable, but we manage. We try to dwell on what we are and can do as a family rather than what we are not and cannot do. I think we have a tremendous amount for which to be thankful. One day, we hope that Alex will outgrow the effects of his run-in with the *E. coli* bacteria. We also hope that someday, before it's too late, we will better understand the origins of his seizure disorder and how to control it. But those thoughts are wishes and we are realists—we recognize that sometimes wishes come true, and sometimes they don't.

And What About the Future?

One of the most difficult things for us to comprehend is the future. In many ways, we don't really think we've hit the hard part yet. Today, it is fundamentally a question of how *we* deal with Alex's medical condition, for like many other kids his age, Alex is still too young to manage his own medical needs. As he gets older and more independent, all of that will change, and, frankly, that can be a very frightening thought.

A number of years ago, I taught at Bucknell University. I had a young student working with me who had been a diabetic since the age of nine. Pam was bright and hard-working and enjoyed life to the fullest. Every weekend she was off on another adventure—rock climbing, skiing, sailing, or spelunking. I first discovered Pam was a diabetic when she came into my office one day, upset about a statement made by her physiological psychology professor during class. They were discussing how insulin works and without thinking about what he was saying or to whom he was saying it, he said point-blank that most childhood diabetics would be dead by the age of twenty.

Well, there she was sitting in the audience. Pam had a very clear idea of her life expectancy, the odds, and what she was up against, but she really resented the way it was said and the fact that it was said in front of her classmates. I remember her sitting in the rocking chair in my office telling me her entire medical history. At the time, I really didn't know what to say, but somehow I managed to give her the comfort she needed. I told her honestly that I really couldn't relate to her medical condition, but I assured her I was there for her in any way she needed. Now, nearly fifteen years later, I finally understand how tough it must have been for her.

The following summer, Pam joined me and a group of students who traveled to New Orleans to study zoo research methodology at the Audubon Zoological Park. More than any of the other students in the group, Pam adopted a "work hard, party hard" mentality, which worried me a bit. But I decided to treat her as an adult capable of managing her own affairs. Although she was ten years my junior, I suspect she had a better understanding of what life was all about than I.

The morning after her graduation, Pam came by to say goodbye. She told me she and a friend had climbed to the top of the water tower on campus in the early hours of the morning—something she had always wanted to do, and something I never would have even considered doing. The tower was at least 150 feet tall, and just the thought of what she had done made me dizzy. She went off to the University of Montana for graduate studies in animal behavior and got involved in a research project tracking the movement of grizzly bears. It was exactly what she wanted to do.

The summer after her first year in graduate school, I got a letter from Pam's mother informing me that her daughter had slipped into a diabetic coma and died. I was stunned. The letter was sweet and informative, thanking me for being such a positive influence on her daughter. Between the lines, I sensed a mother affected as profoundly by the death of her child as by her inability to do anything to prevent it. I still have some pictures of Pam taken at the zoo. In one, she is kneeling next to a tapir, hugging it as if it were her family dog. Her eyes are radiant and her face is bronzed with the tan she worked on like an art. She hid her medical condition well. Only now that I have a son with a life-threatening seizure disorder can I understand what Pam was really all about. I only hope that Alex can live his life to the fullest as she did, although, in all honesty, I hope he will be a little less adventurous. When I opened the letter from Pam's mother years ago, I never imagined that one day I would be a mother, too, and share the same pain over my inability to protect my child forever.

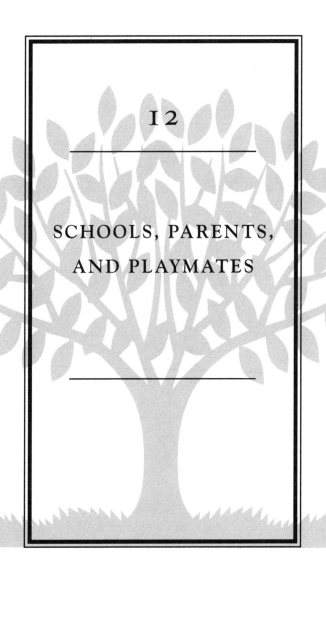

12

SCHOOLS, PARENTS,
AND PLAYMATES

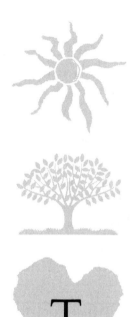

The thought of managing Alex's medical condition at a public school was a daunting one for Tom and me as well as the school's staff. As this book is written, Alex begins kindergarten. Six months of preparation have preceded him. Karen, Alex's pediatrician, and I have trained the entire staff of the school—from the principal to the bus drivers—on how to handle Alex's medical condition. We have an emergency plan in place, with clear written directions on what to do, whom to call, and when to take action. There is an oxygen tank and a pediatric mask on the premises at all times, and Tom and I have made plans to be close by in the event Ativan must be administered. From the time we pre-registered Alex in the school, we began to hear reports that the staff was particularly apprehensive about dealing with a child like Alex. Their anxiety was intensified a bit when a psychologist prescreening

Alex for kindergarten included in his written report: "The team must address several issues. The first is the anxiety of working with a child with a potentially life-threatening condition."

I totally understood their anxiety. For the most part, all they knew about Alex was what they had read on paper. I'm sure that contained just enough information to unnerve even the most experienced educator. We are actually quite fortunate the school is taking Alex's medical condition seriously. It would have troubled us a lot more if they had dismissed our medical concerns with, "Oh, well, so he has seizures. We've dealt with a number of children who have seizures." We decided to address the staff's fears directly: to make sure they were properly trained, to give them a forum to ask questions, and to give them an opportunity to interact with Alex beforehand as a way of alleviating their anxiety.

Alex's bout with the E. *coli* bug and all of his medical problems since that time made Tom and me rethink whether we wanted to live on the top of a mountain, forty-five minutes from the nearest emergency room. A number of close calls and a half-dozen ambulance runs at all hours of the day and night certainly influenced our thinking. It also worried us that Alex would be attending kindergarten in a town that was located fifteen minutes from the nearest rescue squad, and that it would then take another thirty minutes by ambulance to the hospital. We knew it was time to let go and permit him to attend kindergarten on his own (we had already held him back a year), but we also knew that a grand mal seizure at school could have potentially devastating consequences for him.

A year after the E. *coli* infection, we began our search for a place to live within fifteen minutes of the nearest hospital in Brattleboro. We had several other conditions also: We wanted to remain in the same school system, and we wanted to be located no more than a mile off a main road. Our search brought us to Marlboro, where Alex had been attending a private preschool for the past three years.

Building an Educational Team

Our desire to remain in the same school system was based not only on the quality of the schools, but also on the educational team that had been put in place to work with Alex in preschool. The special education program for the school district was run by a parent-oriented director, who was a mother of a special needs child herself. It was the director who first suggested that we have Karen as Alex's pediatrician. That suggestion alone has had an incredible influence on how we cope with Alex's illness. Alex's entire educational team—his case manager, his teachers, his occupational, speech, and physical therapists, and Tom and I—have worked tremendously hard at coordinating his educational needs, ferreting out resources, balancing differences of opinion, and making sure that all of our voices are heard. In short, Alex's educational team has many of the same qualities as the medical team that saved his life.

While Alex was at Dartmouth-Hitchcock Medical Center, nearing the end of his two-month hospital stay from the *E. coli* infection, Alex's case manager, Claire, came to visit and ask how the school system could help in his rehabilitation. When I think about it, that was an incredibly amazing event—like an insurance company asking you how they can help you pay your hospital bills. The pre-kindergarten medical training Alex's pediatrician and I did at the Marlboro Elementary School was Claire's idea. During our semiannual team meeting on Alex's educational needs, we had been discussing Alex's transition to kindergarten when Claire, who was running the meeting, turned to me and asked, "What are your biggest concerns for Alex at this time?" I didn't really plan to say it—I hadn't really even thought about it—but my voice cracked as I answered, "Keeping Alex alive until he gets to kindergarten." Then I couldn't hold my feelings back anymore and I broke down crying. As a result, Alex's educational team remains as concerned about his medical health as his educational plan.

SOME THOUGHTS ON WORKING EFFECTIVELY WITH SCHOOLS

I recently went to a lecture on advocating for your child in the school system. It was presented by a professional who spoke from experience as the mother of a retarded son. For a moment, I felt like I was in the wrong church service, for the advocacy tips all focused on adversarial relationships with the school system. One of the suggestions was to position yourself at team meetings, sitting between people of power. "Wait a minute," I thought. "I hold the position of power at the table, not anyone else. It's my kid's education and my kid's life we're discussing. Why else would we be sitting around the table together?"

The attitude that we hold the power is one that Tom and I have maintained all along, and I think it is one of the reasons we have been able to deal successfully with the school system thus far. *If you have a child with a medical condition, parental involvement is just as important in the school setting as it is in the hospital setting. The more you demonstrate how much you care, the more attention your child receives.* The worst thing you can possibly do is just sit back in a helpless role and assume that the school knows what's best for your child. They don't. You do—because you are the parent.

After I got past the apparently opposite experiences the lecturer on advocacy and I had with our respective school systems, I learned a lot of useful tips, some of which I will paraphrase here along with my thoughts:

Remember that you are your child's best advocate. Be a confident and assertive team player. Know your rights, and make sure everyone understands that you expect to be a critical member of your child's educational team.

Educate yourself on your child's educational needs. Make sure you understand the educational requirements of your child's medical condition or disability. Don't simply accept the school system's point of view. Research your child's educational requirements by talking to social workers, education specialists, psychologists, your physician, and other parents. For example, Alex was recently diagnosed in a school psychological evaluation as having ADHD (attention deficit and hyperactivity disorder), which isn't all that surprising given the head traumas he's experienced. But we didn't simply accept the diagnosis and the recommended educational plan. We researched the latest information on the condition so that we could better evaluate the educational plan.

Never be afraid to ask questions. Ask as many questions as you need to feel comfortable that you understand what is being said. If you are intimidated by asking questions in a group setting, write them down and discuss them later in private with your case manager or advocate.

Take all the time you need to make your point. Try not to get frustrated if you cannot get your point across, and don't let yourself be hurried. If necessary, ask for an additional meeting.

Keep detailed records of meetings and conversations. Take notes on what was said and by whom it was said. You may need to refer back to these notes at a later time to clarify responsibilities or to make a point.

Keep your child and his or her educational needs as the topic of all team meetings. Don't let meetings stray from the topic—discussions of funding availability and experiences with other children are irrelevant to the discussion of your child's needs. For example, suppose you are discussing the need for your child to be tutored in reading skills over the summer. Suddenly, someone starts to tell you there is no money in the school budget. End that conversation by saying: "We're not here to discuss the school budget. We're here to decide whether my child qualifies for the summer reading program."

If some of these tips sound a lot like those useful in dealing with your child's medical team, don't be surprised. In many ways, *the issues involved in healing your child and educating your child are quite similar. Both healing and schooling best occur in a team environment, in which you, the parent, are an essential player.* No one person has all the answers. *The combined views of many professionals and parents, if managed appropriately, can create an ideal environment for growth, whether it be healing or learning related.* When your child experiences a serious injury or illness, it is important to realize that healing goes well beyond recovery. It extends deeply into your child's world, which in most cases involves some sort of schooling environment. How your child views him- or herself and how he or she is accepted by others will have a long-term effect on your child's social, emotional, and intellectual well-being.

SCHOOL IS NOT JUST EDUCATION, IT'S PARENTS AND CLASSMATES, TOO

More than anything else, other parents want to know whether your child's medical condition is contagious. And it's often the case that parents who are uninformed about your child's illness are the most paranoid and are most likely to leap to erroneous conclusions. On many levels, you can't blame them, for all they are doing is looking after the health of their own children. If they don't have any information to the contrary, it's natural to assume a defensive stance. In the case of Alex's seizure disorder, it is easy for other parents to categorize his illness as a neurological condition and view it as nonthreatening. However, when Alex was first diagnosed with the *E. coli* bacterial infection, it was a totally different matter.

IT'S A PUBLIC HEALTH ISSUE

The morning in the emergency room when Alex's pediatrician, Karen, informed us that Alex's stool culture was growing out as *E. coli* 0157:H7, she also asked in a hushed tone whether we understood that it was a public health issue. We didn't, but we soon found out what that meant. She immediately notified the Vermont Department of Health, who in turn notified the Centers for Disease Control in Atlanta. What we first thought was an isolated illness in a matter of hours became a national statistic and potential health crisis. Although on some level we knew we were the victims, not the cause, it still made us feel contaminated. After all, it was a highly virulent strain of bacteria originating (as best we understand) from cow manure or human fecal matter.

At the time, Alex and Marty were attending a summer preschool program in Brattleboro. Alex had been at school only two days before, so Karen suggested I call the school to notify them of Alex's illness and to inquire whether there were any other children showing symptoms of bloody diarrhea. I stood at the desk in the emergency room and made the call. It was not easy to call and say, "Hi, I'm in the emergency room with Alex, who is dying of an *E. coli* bacterial infection, and your entire school might have been exposed." I got the director on the phone, whose reaction was a mixture of heartfelt empathy for Alex and controlled panic.

Then the calls began as the state epidemiologist began tracking the path of Alex's illness. It was like a hurricane upgraded to a Class IV storm headed directly our way. She left several messages on our answering machine as well as at Dartmouth for when we finally arrived. She needed to talk to us immediately to ask questions. Suddenly, our life of anonymity in the country was put under a microscope and broadcast everywhere. Had Alex eaten ground beef or drunk apple cider? Where did we buy our groceries? Where had we been in the last five days? Had we eaten in a restaurant? Had we been near a farm or cows? Where did we live? What was our water supply? Was anyone else in the family sick? Had anyone else we knew been sick? And on and on the questions went.

State health investigators visited our grocery store, the pizza restaurant where we had eaten lunch, and a goat farmer whose baby goat Alex had hugged at a farmer's market. They visited our house for samples of our well water and the water in the stream running behind our house. They even tried to collect stool samples from the squirrels that left droppings on our back deck where the kids played. Our weekend neighbors heard about Alex and made their own calls to the Department of Health, insisting that the water supply around our home must be contaminated. More investigators arrived. Had we not been in the hospital, obsessed with Alex's condition from minute to minute, I'm sure we would have been hysterical with all the investigations going on around us.

We were no longer just familiar faces around town; we were now labeled "the family with the boy with the *E. coli* infection." For months afterward, it was difficult to go out without being paranoid that people were looking and pointing at us. As Alex fought for his life at Dartmouth and then in Boston, the investigation went on, but neither the source of the *E. coli* nor other cases could be identified. It went down on the books as "an isolated case in southern Vermont" and ended at that. But for those families with young children who knew us, it didn't end at all. It was a chilling thought for them to realize that it could have been their children and, worse yet, that the source could still be lurking somewhere in our environment.

Help and Healing of Other Parents

If you've gone through what we've been through, you've probably learned that other parents can be a great source of help in managing your child's medical concerns. Even after Alex recovered from the bacterial infection and could talk and walk again, his pediatrician wanted him to wait another month before returning to school. She felt he had little reserves and was worried that if he contracted a virus, it would set his recovery back for months. We, too, were worried and spent the month totally avoiding any places where he might come into contact with sick people or other children.

When Alex finally went back to school, we made sure the staff and other parents understood the precariousness of Alex's health and the importance of not sending their children to school if they were sick. At the time, I thought about sending a letter to the other parents outlining our concerns over Alex's health. I've included the letter I wrote, but never sent, because I was able to talk with each of the other parents individually. But if you live in a well-populated area and your child attends a large school, you might want to send a letter like the following:

Dear Parent,

My son Alex attends preschool with your child. Last summer he contracted a serious bacterial infection and was hospitalized for two months. He has recovered from the immediate effects of the illness and he is not contagious. However, the illness has left him with a life-threatening seizure disorder. Any minor illness involving a fever or a virus, such as the chicken pox, may have very serious consequences for him.

Because of this, I would appreciate knowing if your child is exposed to or has contracted chicken pox. I would also appreciate knowing if your child has any other fever-related illness to which Alex has been exposed. The information you provide will allow us to adjust Alex's medication levels to minimize the effects of any illness.

Please feel free to call me with questions. Thank you for helping Alex through this difficult time.

Sincerely,

Nancy Cain

Maybe it was luck or maybe it was the combined efforts of the other families, but Alex never caught a virus from school. One mother did call me when her son was diagnosed with strep throat and possibly viral meningitis. Alex had a cough and a runny nose, so our pediatrician immediately put him on antibiotics as a precaution. Alex did get the chicken pox one summer and ended up in the hospital just like we expected, but it was Marty who appeared to be the culprit. We never did figure out where Marty caught it.

THE HEALING POWER OF PLAYMATES

Children appear to be able to heal other children in a way that we as parents can't begin to do. I guess that is because a child in some way takes his or her parents' love for granted, but when unconditional love comes from a peer, it is perceived as something truly special. Alex has a friend, named Whitney, who did a lot for his spirits following his bout with *E. coli* and his colostomy-reversal surgery. In particular, I remember picking Alex up from the school's play yard one warm spring day. Alex was sitting on the little hill in the yard talking and holding hands with Whitney.

When I walked up, Whitney popped up with her dark curls literally bouncing and announced, "Me and Alex are the same. We both had op-ray-shuns," which she pronounced very seriously and deliberately. Then she tugged on her leggings to show me the site where she had undergone surgery for removal of a cyst. Alex responded by pushing his sock down and showing off the large crinkly scar on his ankle. They were beaming with pride, which I thought was a truly wonderful way to deal with the medical wounds they had both endured. I also thought it was interesting that Alex chose to display the scar on his ankle, not the ones from his more recent abdominal surgery. I wondered if he was revealing the wound that was easier for both him and her to understand. Until I stumbled on that scene, I don't think I had thought much about the role other children played in Alex's physical, mental, and spiritual healing.

I observed a very positive encounter between Alex and Whitney. I credit her mother with explaining Whitney's and Alex's medical problems in a way that young children could understand. Clearly Whitney felt pretty good about herself and her surgery. We, too, had been working very hard to make Alex feel good about himself, but it was Whitney who did wonders for his self-esteem.

The Negative Side of Peers

Peer encounters following a critical illness or injury can just as easily be devastating and significantly undermine the healing process. Particularly if a child shows some effect of the illness, be it hair loss, visible scars, or in the case of Alex, an ostomy bag hanging from his belly, it can be disarming to other children. Children who don't understand and who are frightened by another's physical appearance can be unusually cruel. I know. I was once one of them.

Barbara's Braces

When I was in fifth grade, a new girl moved into our class. In the small town where I grew up, a new kid alone was an unusual event, but the fact that this girl was about a foot shorter than the rest of us and wore leg braces made her truly unusual. Our teacher introduced Barbara to the class, but never told us she had polio as a young child. We learned that from Barbara herself, but because it wasn't explained, it didn't mean much to us. What we did understand was this new girl was now getting all of the teacher's attention. Previously, I had been the top student in the class and had earned the unofficial designation of teacher's pet. Now I had been pushed aside by this miniature girl with leg braces, who happened to be a good student as well.

I was angry, and my best friend, Judy, was angry, too. We were never directly cruel to Barbara other than deliberately ignoring her, but we devised our own way to deal with our discomfort. Judy brought a Barbie doll to school, which we dressed up like Barbara and outfitted with a set of leg braces made out of bent paper clips. We hid the doll under the radiator in the girls' bathroom and sneaked into the school during recess and acted out all sorts of dramas with the doll as if she were Barbara herself. They weren't nice dramas either. We were obsessed with Barbara because she threatened us and we simply did not understand her or her medical condition.

If someone, either our teacher or Barbara's parents, had taken the time to explain her illness to us, it would have made Barbara's adjustment to the school much smoother. It would also have prevented the fear and resentment that children like me developed. I am thankful that schools and teachers today are far more progressive and sensitive to issues such as these, particularly since my son Alex has become the "Barbara" of his class.

As a parent, you can do a tremendous amount for your children. You can bathe them in love, comfort them, and encourage them. But you can't make other children like them, accept them, and want to share their toys with them. This causes a lot of anxiety for parents like me who have children with medical conditions. I know I can't build Alex's social relationships for him, but I feel it is my responsibility as a parent to try to ensure that his classmates understand his medical condition in a nonpejorative and nonthreatening way. How do you do this? If your child is not old enough to explain his or her own illness, either the teacher must educate the students or the parents must educate their children. As Alex's parent, my role is that of training the trainer—be it the teacher or the parents of Alex's classmates—and it is a far from easy role.

TRAINING THE TRAINER

Of course, the extent to which you can educate school staff members, other parents, and their children depends on the nature of the school system and their attitude toward children with special needs and medical conditions. My experience, which is confirmed by the experience of many others, is that individual staff members will often go out of their way to help you and your child if you approach your child's classroom needs from a team perspective. For example, if you ask for help in making your child's adaptation to the classroom the least disruptive for your child and his or her classmates, you are likely to get a great deal of support. If on the other hand you expect the classroom (teacher and students included) to adapt to your child, you are likely to run into obstacles. The healing that goes on between two people, be it physician and patient or one child with another, requires mutual understanding and the desire of both parties to participate in the healing process. In general, I'm an optimist. I don't think most people want to be uncooperative or obstructionist; I think they get that way when they are not informed or are otherwise threatened.

TRAINING THE TEACHER

One of the most important things you can provide for teachers and staff members is a written summary of your child's medical history. This summary should be written by you, the parent, in language the school will understand. A summary like this gives a teacher a far better understanding of your child's medical condition and allows him or her to read it and think about its contents. If you simply describe the history of your child's illness in person, you run the risk of the listener focusing on one aspect and not hearing the rest of what you have to say. You might wonder why you can't simply send along medical records from your physicians. There are two important reasons to write this document yourself: First, you can emphasize aspects of your child's illness that you think merit attention and deemphasize those you do not. Second, a teacher will respond far more personally and will have a greater sense of involvement in a description written in your own words.

I recently wrote Alex's medical history for the school nurse and the staff at Marlboro Elementary School. It was nearly five typed pages. If that seems like a lot, imagine how lengthy Alex's official medical records would be if I included all the information from the eight different hospitals he's been in (some a half-dozen or more times) in five different states. Just a listing of the metabolic tests he's undergone reads like a chapter out of a chemistry textbook. No one could begin to make sense of this myriad of medical records. In my summary, I started with his birth and highlighted only those critical events that made him what he is today. It's important for the school staff to understand who he is, but I think it is even more important for them to understand where he is going.

Once you have given a copy of your child's medical history to the school staff, you need to give them the opportunity to understand its contents. When you schedule a meeting to discuss your child and his or her illness, there are a number of other questions you might want to ask the teacher:

How will you explain my child's illness (or medical condition) to the other children? This is an essential question to ask, for it also tells you how well the teacher understands your child and gives you the opportunity to correct any misunderstandings. You can also take this opportunity to make any suggestions that you feel appropriate.

How will you involve my child in your answers? Will the teacher have your child help explain his or her illness? Will the teacher discuss your child's illness privately with the other students? These are things you will probably have an opinion about, and it is better to know up front how the teacher will approach questions by other students.

How will you explain my child's illness to other parents? Your child's classmates will undoubtedly mention your child at home and may ask their parents about your child's condition. The teacher needs to be prepared to discuss your child's illness and medical needs with other parents. If in fact you find that the teacher is getting a lot of questions from parents, you might want to offer to meet directly with them. I think there is nothing better than a good parent-to-parent chat to dispel any fears and to elicit the support of other parents in your child's classroom adaptation.

You can also do your child a lot of good by collecting or suggesting reading materials for the classroom that help others understand your child. I can tell you from experience that Marty has had an almost insatiable need to understand Alex's hospitalization and his ongoing seizure disorder. In general, I have to say that "issues" books (e.g., a book on a turtle who has epilepsy) have elicited more questions from Marty than they have provided explanations. Both

Alex and Marty seem to want to understand more than how a character deals with an illness, so we have also read them books on hospitalization and medicine as well as books on the inner workings of the body and the mind.

One book, in particular, called *Going to the Hospital*, features Mr. Rogers and has been very comforting to Alex. It is not at all unusual for me to find Alex sitting quietly in the family room with the book open in his lap studying the pictures. Obviously, the most appropriate books for your child depend on your child's situation and age. The Association for the Care of Children's Health is a good place to start your search for reading materials. It publishes an annotated bibliography of books on hospitalization, illness, and disabling conditions for children of all ages (write ACCH, 7910 Woodmont Avenue, Suite 300, Bethesda, Maryland 20814; 301-654-6549).

Training Other Parents

Dealing with other parents can be a tricky matter. The first thing you realize is that you can't control what parents tell their children or how children interpret what they hear. A friend of mine, who has a four-year-old with special needs, recently told me a story illustrating just that point. Her son attends a private preschool under a federally mandated, state-administered program that provides free preschool tuition for children with special needs. One day when a classmate of her son's came over to play, the boy announced, "My daddy says you don't pay your bills." My friend was stunned to hear such an accusation from a four-year-old. She felt silly being embarrassed, but found herself defensively denying the accusation, telling him that she certainly did pay her bills. The scene bothered her for some time until she figured out where it had come from—her son's classmate had either been told or had overheard his parents talking about the fact that her son didn't pay any preschool tuition.

Because you can't control what parents tell their children or how children interpret what they hear, the best you can do is make sure that other parents have the facts. As I mentioned earlier, if you are dealing with chronic illness like Alex's seizure disorder, or a child undergoing chemotherapy for leukemia, you might consider writing a letter to other parents after obtaining the approval of school officials. Before sending a letter, make sure the teacher is well educated about your child's illness so that he or she can field any questions that arise. One issue that commonly surfaces is that other children or their parents are troubled by the fact that a child with a medical condition receives special attention. As a parent, it is your responsibility to ensure that your child is not being overprotected in the classroom. At the same time, if your child requires special attention or the services of a classroom aide, make sure other parents understand that it is your child's *illness*, not *your child*, that necessitates the extra attention.

Inevitably, you must explain more details to parents if your child is going over to another child's house to play. Make sure that the parent is comfortable dealing with your child's illness and make sure that he or she understands what to do in the case of an emergency. Other parents, as long as you inform them of what to expect, can help a lot in giving your child a greater sense of independence.

TRAINING YOUR CHILD

Any discussion of how to deal with schools, parents, and playmates wouldn't be complete without emphasizing the necessity of preparing your child to talk about his or her illness. At a most basic level, you must make sure your child knows how to answer questions asked by schoolmates. For example, your child should never have to feel disarmed by a classmate who asks, "Are you going to die?" or "Why do your arms flap when you run?" Even if you have been honest with your child and explained his or her illness in great detail, your child may not know how to answer such a question when it is posed by a peer. Depending on your child's age, give your child the opportunity to "try out" his or her explanations through dramatic play or simply by rehearsing what he or she will say under certain circumstances.

Sometimes I think that preparing Alex to enter the public school system has been like experiencing the helplessness of seeing him so critically ill all over again. We've nursed and nurtured him through a horribly acute illness. And now we're doing the best we can to balance his need for independence with the reality of a life-threatening chronic illness. We've done all this by getting actively involved in his medical care, by making accommodations in our lives for his illness, and by giving him all of the love and encouragement we can. As I write this, I think forward to the first day of school. When he climbs on the school bus at the end of our driveway for the first time, I'm sure I will cry, not because I am sad, but because in many ways I will feel helpless. Tom and I, along with all of the professionals supporting Alex, have done our best to make his transition into the public school system as smooth and safe as possible. But once again, I realize I have to give up some control— I have to pass the ball and trust the team, Alex's educational team—as Alex embarks on another phase of his life.

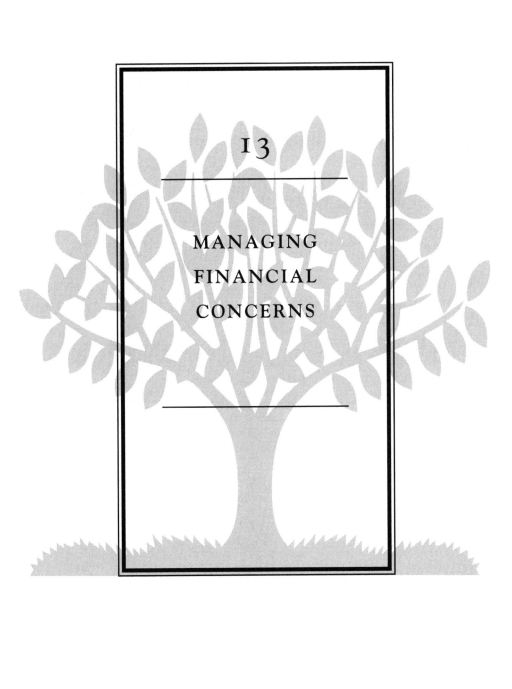

13

MANAGING
FINANCIAL
CONCERNS

stimating the cost of Alex's illness is a lot like assessing the damage of a hurricane. You can't place a value on a lifetime of memories or dashed hopes for the future. You can only speak of the financial cost—the cost to rebuild and to begin again. We never imagined the tremendous amount of medical resources, approximately $315,000 worth, that would be required to sustain Alex's life and to get him to where he is today. And those were just the medical costs. Beneath the medical bills were many hidden costs—the costs not covered by medical insurance, the cost of disrupting our careers, and the cost of living in limbo for months on end. What we didn't know at first was that there are sources of financial support available to help families like ours. Many institutions, organizations, and governmental agencies

have programs that provide various forms of financial support. You just need to know how to ask for them.

This was something we first discovered when Alex was at Children's Hospital in Boston. Alex had been in the hospital nearly two weeks before we discovered the social services department. We found it down some out-of-the-way corridor after asking three different people for directions. I hesitantly walked in and told the receptionist that a cashier in the cafeteria said we should come and get some meal tickets. In a few minutes, a social worker came out and asked me a few questions about Alex's medical condition and how long he had been in the hospital. He thought we might be eligible for meal tickets and told us to come back later in the day after he had reviewed Alex's hospital records.

We returned that afternoon and were given a book of twenty-eight dollars for a week's worth of meals. For every week Alex was hospitalized, we were told to return for another book. I was totally surprised to find that eligibility was based on length of stay rather than pure financial need. I was amazed to find that we were eligible for free parking in the hospital's garage as well. We had been spending six dollars a day, and the cost was beginning to add up. Our encounter in the social services department also led to the discovery that the hospital had subsidized housing for parents, and we put ourselves on the waiting list. Up to this point, we had been staying in the hospital's parents' lounge. Since we had been told that Alex would probably be in Boston for at least two months, we knew it was time to start looking for some more permanent housing.

THE QUESTION OF FINANCES

The question of finances is always of foremost concern for parents who suddenly find their child seriously ill or injured. The most basic question is, do you have medical insurance? If you don't, you can't help but wonder whether your child's medical treatment will be compromised for economic reasons, either by your inability to pay or by the hospital's de facto policies concerning uninsured patients. Within the first half hour of admittance to every one of the six emergency rooms in which Alex has been treated, we were visited by a hospital administrator carrying a clipboard who asked, "How are you going to pay for this?" We are fortunate that we have medical insurance and could always answer with the name of our insurer. But, if you don't have insurance, this is the time to ask, "Will my child be treated any differently because I am not insured?" If you don't get a satisfactory answer, make sure you ask to speak with a hospital social worker—it is his or her job to help you work out a mutually acceptable way to cover the costs of hospitalization.

In a medical crisis, you do what you have to do without regard to the financial cost. But it is not long before you begin to think about how you're going to handle the situation financially. Even with medical insurance, you will find yourself asking many questions: How broad is my insurance coverage? Do I have to pay any deductibles? Is there a cap on the claims my insurer will pay? Will there be treatments that my insurance will not cover? For example, following Alex's hospitalization with the *E. coli* infection, it was recommended that he go to a rehabilitation facility, but our HMO would not pay for it. Instead, he stayed in the hospital a week longer and was sent home with a feeding tube in his nose, surgical dressings for his ankle, and clear instructions on how to administer various forms of physical and occupational therapy. For weeks after, Tom and I spent most of our days and nights acting as Alex's nurses and rehabilitation therapists.

As soon as you can get a copy of your medical insurance policy, take the time to review it to make sure you understand your coverage. If there is anything you don't understand, don't hesitate to call your insurer for an explanation. Whatever you do, you don't want to find out after the fact that you have violated some tiny clause in your medical insurance policy that leaves you liable for a great deal of your child's hospitalization costs. You also will want to know ahead of time what your insurance won't cover once you leave the hospital. We discovered, for example, that our HMO would pay for the cost of Alex's colostomy surgery, but would not pay for his colostomy supplies on an outpatient basis. After looking at the ridiculous cost of ostomy bags, ostomy wafers, protective oint-ments, sealants, and the like, we discovered it was going to cost us nearly $200 a month. We didn't have a choice, but it was some-thing we knew we had to include in our monthly budget.

No less of a financial concern than your insurance coverage is the impact of your child's injury or illness on your job. Can you af-ford to take unpaid leave from your job in order to spend time with your child? Will the time you spend with your child have a long-term effect on your career or job stability? If you own your own business, can you afford to take time off with your child? If so, who will run your business in your absence? In our situation, I had to call my new editor, with whom I had just signed a contract the day before Alex came down with the bacterial infection. I had to tell her I couldn't make the deadline we had just negotiated. Luckily, she was an extraordinarily understanding and compassionate per-son—it was nearly six months before I was able to write again.

THE HIDDEN COSTS OF HOSPITALIZATION

When Alex was first hospitalized with the *E. coli* infection, we naively thought that his illness would not have much of a financial impact on us. How wrong we were. Within minutes of arriving in the emergency room in Brattleboro, it was obvious that he had to be transferred to a regional medical center for pediatric surgery. Suddenly, we were at Dartmouth-Hitchcock Medical Center, nearly two hours from home. Now we had commuting costs, temporary housing costs, higher meal costs, and the costs of maintaining our home while we were away. When his condition worsened and his kidneys failed, he was transferred even farther away to Boston Children's Hospital for pediatric dialysis.

In a large metropolitan city, three hours from home, our costs skyrocketed. We had been staying at a home for parents and families of hospitalized children near Dartmouth called David's House for $10 a night. Breakfast had been provided for free, and we were able to cook our own meals. In Boston, there was a similar facility called Ronald McDonald House nearby. But it was not available to us, for it was limited to families of children with cancer. The best we could do for housing, aside from camping out in the parents' lounge, was to live in the subsidized hotel next door for $50 a night. Between housing, meals, parking, and commuting costs, we suddenly found ourselves spending nearly $80 a day to live. It didn't take us long to figure out that we were looking at a cost of nearly $5,000 just to live in Boston for the next two months!

It was not only an emotional relief to see Alex finally sent home, but also a financial relief. I remember our first night home together as a family. Marty was so pleased to be back in his room again, but he was afraid to be alone in the dark. We set Alex up in our bed and attached a bag of liquid diet to the bedpost like an IV. As he slept, we fed him through the feeding tube in his nose. We were afraid to take our eyes off him for even a minute. Within days of being home, we realized that the cost of his hospitalization was being supplanted by the cost of his recovery. It seemed like we were in a pharmacy or doctor's office nearly every day, getting prescriptions, filling prescriptions, buying more Ensure (a complete liquid diet at a cost of $2 a can or $6 a day) or more Polycose (a powdered caloric additive at $8 a can). Every once in a while, the UPS truck would arrive with another box of ostomy supplies and an invoice of several hundred dollars inside. The cost of his recovery was far less than our living costs during his hospitalization, but the out-of-pocket costs not covered by insurance still came to over $400 a month.

As Alex's illness and recovery lingered, Tom returned to his consulting work out of necessity, since we were really beginning to feel the loss of income. I assumed the role of Alex's at-home nurse and health care provider. We were at home again, but we were really kidding ourselves if we thought we were out of the hospital. Many a day and night we were on the phone with Alex's pediatrician in Brattleboro or his neurologist at Dartmouth—Alex's breathing was labored, Alex was vomiting up his liquid formula, or Alex was showing seizurelike movements in his sleep. But slowly we nursed him back to health. His ankle wound healed, his ostomy site grew less irritated, his feeding tube was removed, he began to tolerate more solid foods, and he began again to use the muscles of his arms and legs that had been dormant for over two months. We packed the feeding tubes, the feeding bags, the stethoscope, the surgical gauze, the surgical tape, and all the other medical paraphernalia we'd acquired into a box and put it in the closet. But it was nearly a year and over $5,000 more of out-of-pocket expenses before Alex recovered enough to have his colon reattached and to eat normal food without costly nutritional supplements.

Hidden Forms of Support

We were overwhelmed by the hidden costs of Alex's illness—the hidden costs of his hospitalization as well as his recovery. At first, we rejected offers of financial support from our families, but as time went on, we swallowed our pride and accepted them. It was their way of trying to help us from afar, and it gave us one less stressful thing to deal with. We found ourselves in the position of many others when it comes to the high cost of things like health care and education. It appeared that we had too many resources to qualify for federal or state assistance programs, but not enough disposable income to weather the financial impact of a catastrophic illness like Alex's. We also learned, though, that it was wrong to assume we were not eligible for any form of financial support. Out there, through the good graces of individuals and foundations, and little-known waivers for special situations, there is a significant amount of hidden financial support for children with serious illnesses, injuries, or medical concerns.

It is impossible to enumerate the various sources of financial support available because they vary from institution to institution and from state to state. For example, Children's Hospital in Boston, through various benefactors, had a broad program of financial support, including subsidies for housing, parking, and meals. Dartmouth-Hitchcock Medical Center, on the other hand, had provided low-cost (or free if you could not afford to pay) housing in a homelike environment to every family of ill or injured children. Sometimes we were told about the financial support available. Other times, we had to figure it out on our own or have a friendly cashier bring it to our attention.

A social worker at Children's Hospital told us about Supplemental Social Security payments that Alex was eligible for under Section XVI of the Social Security Act. Although our family did not meet the SSI (supplemental security income) guidelines, Alex became eligible after spending one calendar month at Children's Hospital. Under the provisions of the law, when a child is institutionalized (e.g., in an intermediate care facility or a hospital), only the child's, and not the parents', income is considered in determining SSI eligibility. Called a Waiver of Parental Deeming, it is provided for by Section 1614(F)(2) of Social Security Act Regulations 416.1160-1169 and 416.1202-1204a. The social worker guided us through the maze of paperwork and coached us on how to fill out the forms. I don't think we ever would have figured out that a program like that existed on our own.

We also found some more long-term financial assistance from the state of Vermont's Division of Children with Special Health Care Needs. It has no arbitrary cutoff for assistance. Rather, it bases its support on cost-sharing and a sliding scale of income. I mention this program only because it illustrates the type of program that might be out there in your state, municipality, or county. Finding, rather than qualifying for, programs such as these is the challenge.

How do you find out about programs like these? The first and best place to ask is your state health department or a local parent-to-parent organization. All fifty states currently have parent-to-parent organizations or similar organizations that serve as parent support groups and information clearinghouses for parents of children with special health needs or disabilities. If you have difficulty locating your local organization, try contacting the following organization for referral information: National Parent-to-Parent Support and Information System, Inc., P.O. Box 907, Blue Ridge, Georgia 30513; 800-651-1151.

Some of the financial support we received also came with a great deal of love attached. There were "love gifts" of cash given to us by the Loose Knit Group of West Dover's Congregational Church, and gifts of money from total strangers, who were touched in some way by Alex's illness. One Sunday while Alex was in Boston, Tom returned to Vermont and attended church. In the fellowship gathering after church, an anonymous man pressed a $100 bill into Tom's hand and disappeared. Tom was so taken off guard that he didn't even get the man's name. Nor did he get a good look at him, save the single detail that the man was wearing a Grateful Dead T-shirt. When we arrived home, six inches of hospital bills were piled up waiting for us. Just about the time I was wondering what I was supposed to do with all of them, the phone rang, and it was our representative from Community Health Plan (CHP), our insurer. We didn't know her—we were only one subscriber among thousands. She was just calling us to let us know how sorry she was for what had happened to Alex and to tell us that she had instructed the claims department to cover *all* the hospital charges. "Just ignore all the bills you get in the mail," she told us. "The last thing you need is more stress." We were astonished by the graciousness of our insurer. It illustrated for us the fact that people really do want to help out in circumstances such as ours.

Long-term Financial Support: Who in the World Is Katie Beckett?

When your child has a chronic or ongoing medical condition, the financial issues become far more stressful. For us, it seems like the end is never in sight. We are fortunate that our medical insurer does not have a lifetime cap on medical expenses (yet), although we recognize that the issue of capitation is being widely discussed as a way of controlling future medical costs of an ever-aging population. It is a very disturbing thought to parents like us, for it is implicitly putting a dollar value on our child's life. For example, if my insurer has a lifetime cap of $500,000, is that the worth of Alex's life?

Given the high cost of medical insurance and the issue of capitation looming ahead, it gives us a little comfort to know that there are some long-term sources of financial support available for children with medical impairments and other disabilities. For those who qualify, Medicaid has a program to cover disabled children. But for those who don't qualify for Medicaid on an income or resource basis, many states allow you to apply for a Medicaid option regardless of the parents' income. In Vermont and some other states, it is known as the "Katie Beckett Waiver" or the Disabled Children Home Care (DCHC) Option. A number of states currently subscribe to the federal Medicaid program. To determine if your state has such a program, contact your State Department of Health, and ask about their Children with Special Health Care Needs programs (which are funded through Title V of the Social Security Act).

The Katie Beckett option is not something that is advertised on posters in the subway or billboards along the highway. In fact, if you never have any reason to be in a Medicaid office, you could go a lifetime without hearing about it. Despite Alex's long medical history, it was only in the past year that it was first mentioned to me by Alex's early education coordinator. It sounded like a source of financial support we should pursue, but the first question I had was, "Who in the world is Katie Beckett?" It took some serious research to discover that Katie Beckett was a three-year-old girl in Iowa, respirator-dependent and paralyzed almost since birth, who was living her life in a hospital because she would lose her Medicaid benefits if she left the hospital. Outside the hospital, her parents' income was above the Medicaid guidelines, but they could not afford the $3,400-a-month cost for home treatment. Instead of living in her home, where she would receive better care, she was costing the taxpayers $12,000 a month to keep her in the hospital. In 1981, President Reagan intervened on her behalf and the then secretary of Health and Human Services granted her a special Medicaid waiver. Since that time, the Medicaid option has been extended to disabled children, eighteen years of age or younger, if it is determined that

- the child requires a level of care provided in a hospital, nursing facility, or intermediate care facility for the mentally retarded;
- the child can be cared for outside an institution;
- home care costs are estimated to be less than institutional costs.

LOTS OF GUILT AND A LEGAL DEFENSE

For several years now, Tom and I have provided a level of care for Alex equivalent to that of a hospital or nursing facility, and I guess it shows. Rarely do we meet a new medical professional who doesn't ask if I am a physician myself. But we had to get over a lot of guilt and trepidation to decide to apply for a Katie Beckett Waiver for Alex. By applying for a Medicaid waiver we were admitting to the world that Alex's medical condition and related problems were truly a disability that wasn't going away. It was a big step for us. Maybe it was our state of mind or maybe it was the process, but from the time we sent in the initial application, it seemed as though we had become players in an absurdist play by Ionesco. Nothing was simple or straightforward. In fact, it seemed to be deliberately complicated.

The first thing that happened was that we received a form letter from the Vermont Department of Social Welfare informing us that Alex was not eligible for Medicaid. It came printed by a dot matrix printer, all in capital letters, on paper that was perforated along the edges. It was one of those impersonal printed letters where the computer fills in the blanks and pretends to type a personalized letter. It reminded me of an IRS communication. The blanks, however, didn't quite match the content. It began:

> TO DETERMINE IF YOU ARE ELIGIBLE FOR BENE-
> FITS OR TO FIGURE OUT THE AMOUNT OF THOSE
> BENEFITS, WE NEED THE FOLLOWING VERIFICA-
> TION (PROOF) OF YOUR SITUATION:

> MR. AND MRS. CAIN, ALEXANDER HAS BEEN
> DENIED MEDICAID UNDER THE KATIE BECKETT
> RULES.

Enclosed with the letter was a notification of "your right to appeal." It said: "You can request a hearing, in person, over the phone, or in writing, if you don't agree with this decision. If you want free legal help, call your local Vermont Legal Aid office which is listed in your telephone book." So, I called the local social services office and informed the caseworker that I wanted to appeal the decision in person. I then asked to whom I was making the appeal. Their lawyers, she answered. The next thing I knew, I had engaged the services of two intelligent and extremely dedicated lawyers with the Vermont Developmental Disabilities Law Project and had begun the process of preparing to appeal the decision. But all along, I couldn't help but wonder why the appeal required the services of lawyers to convince the state that my son had a life-threatening disorder and required twenty-four-hour monitoring. Why wouldn't a simple letter from my pediatrician and/or neurologist be sufficient?

Over the next several months, I met with my lawyers and reviewed every minute detail of Alex's care. We reviewed the law and legal precedents, and we talked through things I had never even thought of before, like, "Who would provide the level of care you do for Alex if something happened to you or Tom?" Finally, the day of the hearing arrived. It was a tense, stressful hour-and-a-half testimony attended by me, my two lawyers, and a state assistant attorney general, and mediated by an impartial hearing officer. I was a bit surprised to find that we were dealing with reasonable people who were sincerely trying to make a fair and well-informed decision.

As I sat there, I realized the tremendous amount of fortitude required to appeal a social services decision. It really made me wonder how many people would take it this far. In all honesty, I don't think I would have, had I known how involved it was and how guilty it would make me feel. No matter how it was presented, I was being put in the position of defending why my child was more needy than another. The faces of other parents with children with far more heart-wrenching disabilities than Alex's kept floating through my mind like demons. I had to keep telling myself that this was a case about Alex and no one else. I had to keep telling myself that I was appealing the decision because it was my right.

I left the hearing with a colossal migraine headache, but at least it was over. Then we waited approximately a month and a half for the decision. One day, a letter came from my lawyer, with a letter from the assistant attorney general attached—it appeared that the state had reversed its earlier decision and granted Alex the Katie Beckett Medicaid waiver. Frankly, I was amazed, but it really did confirm in my mind that we had done the right thing.

It took a lot of energy, both physically and psychologically speaking, to apply for the Medicaid waiver for Alex. I am glad we did it, because I think parents of children with chronic medical conditions need to speak up and fight for their rights. If Alex is accorded certain rights under the law, I don't think bureaucrats (or forms, for that matter) should be able to intimidate me into not exercising them. Should your child qualify for governmental or institutional aid, I encourage you to pursue it, but don't underestimate the stress involved. Investigate the law and be confident of your rights, and as hard as it may be, try not to compare your situation or your child's medical condition to anyone else's.

A Few Final Tips on Managing Financial Concerns

Study your insurance policy for types of coverage before agreeing to treatments and other medical procedures. In a life-and-death situation, the last thing you consider is what it will cost to save your child, and no one expects you to. But as your child becomes more stable, make sure you know what your insurance policy covers. If you find problems, make sure you discuss them. We have found hospitals, medical personnel, and social workers to be both helpful and creative in finding ways to cover all medical costs without compromising our child's care.

Follow carefully the "rules" of your insurer. This may sound like an obvious point, but it is one that shouldn't be overlooked. Many insurance companies and HMOs today control costs by installing certain rules and approval-process requirements in your policy. We are insured by an HMO, for example, that requires that our pediatrician obtain approval for all medical costs, regardless of the provider of services. Even when Alex had to be transferred from Dartmouth-Hitchcock Medical Center to another hospital with pediatric dialysis facilities, the choice of the hospital had to be approved by our HMO through our pediatrician.

Never pay out of pocket. Dealing with medical billing offices, insurance companies, and health care providers can be a daunting task. We've found that the best way to handle the competing voices is to funnel everything through our insurance company, in much the same way as they handle all the medical approvals. We avoid at all costs paying any bills ourselves until we are sure our insurance company has denied them. Once the bill is paid, it is much more difficult to get reimbursed than to have the insurance company work out the billing problem directly with your medical provider. For example, we once got a bill that had been turned over to a collection agency by one of Alex's surgeons who demanded that we pay a shortfall not covered by insurance. Instead of paying the bill, we called our insurer's claims department for an explanation and discovered that the claim had been settled at an agreed-upon amount. Our insurer was outraged to find that we were being held accountable for an additional amount. Had we first paid it, do you think that the surgeon's billing service would have refunded it?

Carry insurance cards and information. More often than not, we have found that our billing problems have resulted from the admitting office of a hospital having incorrect insurance information. We found this particularly to be a problem when Alex required emergency hospitalizations in other states. An Empire Blue Cross–Blue Shield claim of ours once bounced around a number of New York offices for nearly a year until someone got it right. Make a point of carrying your insurance card or at least the policy number in your wallet at all times—you never know when you will need it.

Know your rights and entitlements. Particularly if you are not insured, make sure that you understand your rights and entitlements.

If you have any questions, make sure that you ask to speak with a hospital social worker right away.

Ask about subsidies, hospital programs, etc. Always make a point of asking about hospital programs for financial assistance or meal, housing, and parking subsidies. Often these programs are not advertised. Hospital social workers or hospital social service departments are the best sources of information on this topic.

If necessary, request a discount for air travel. Most airlines have an unpublicized policy of allowing immediate family members to travel at a 50 percent discount off the regular fare in the event of a death in the family or a critical illness. The airlines require "proof" of the death or illness in the form of an obituary or a physician's letter; however, most will allow you to travel to the destination in an emergency and provide the documentation on the return trip. This is a particularly good policy to know about if you need another family member to travel a distance to help out with your child's care.

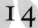

14

FOR EXTENDED FAMILY MEMBERS AND FRIENDS: HOW TO DEAL WITH PARENTS OF ILL OR INJURED CHILDREN

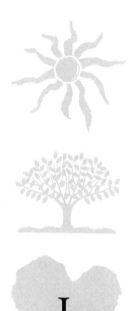

I often feel at a loss to describe how Tom and I felt and how we made it through the critical weeks of Alex's illness. We spent many hours together beside Alex's bed. He was lying inert in a coma, silent and still, but his presence was all around us. It wasn't at all like the old days before we had children, when we would sit and reflect together. The body and soul lying between us had added another dimension to our relationship. It had stretched the boundaries of our love into the infrared range of the spectrum—to a zone you could no longer see, but only feel. At that time, our list of needs seemed endless: from needing a nonjudgmental shoulder to cry on to someone to wash out our socks and underwear for the following day.

As best I can, I would like to tell you my idea of what parents really need at a time like this. Although they may keep you at a distance, for the simple act of communicating with friends and family can itself be exhausting, there is so much you can do to add positive energy to the situation. More than anything, parents need to feel your unqualified love and genuine caring. They don't need your pity, your anger, your fear, or your advice; they need your help.

PARENTS NEED . . .

Time to be alone with each other. As the critical phase of Alex's illness progressed from days to weeks, Tom and I found that we really needed some time alone with each other. On the one hand, we were fearful of leaving Alex by himself. What if he took a sudden turn for the worse? What if he opened his eyes for the first time and was terrified? At the same time, we needed desperately to be out of the hospital environment alone for a few hours, away from the sickness and pathos that surrounded us. But we didn't want to leave Alex with just anyone. We wanted to leave him with the loving and watchful eyes of someone he knew—a close family member or friend with a voice that was familiar and soothing and a touch that said, "You're special to me." One of the greatest gifts you can give to a family with a hospitalized child is your offer to be with the child, not as a visitor, but as a family member the parents can trust.

To know, even from a distance, that you genuinely care. There are many ways you can express your love from afar: by sending cards, books, or little gifts; by organizing prayer groups and offering prayers; by giving blood; or by the act of volunteering to spend some time with another hospitalized child. It didn't matter if we were in the ICU or a hospital room, nearly every day a card or package arrived from my brother Martin and his wife, Cheri. Sometimes they were for us, sometimes they were for Alex, and sometimes they were for Marty, but they always brightened our day. In fact, it was Cheri who opened up my eyes to the true healing potential of parents by sending me Bernie Siegel's book *Love, Medicine and Miracles*. What a gift of love that book was.

A person they can trust to take care of siblings. One of our greatest concerns, particularly during the first week of Alex's illness, was what we were going to do with Marty. We knew we didn't have the physical or emotional energy to deal with him while making many of the critical decisions concerning Alex's illness. We also felt very strongly that *both* of us needed to be with Alex, for Alex's sake as well as each other's. We were lucky that my mother happened to be visiting from South Carolina and that my sister was able to drop everything and come over from Ithaca to help out. By having Marty with people he knew and trusted in his own home, we were able to minimize the amount of stress placed on him and, consequently, on us.

Someone to manage their life on the outside. It always feels like we are miles from home when Alex is in the hospital, and usually we are. Particularly when we were staying in Boston, a three-hour drive from home, it was difficult to take care of all the things going on at home. There were bills to be paid, mail to be gathered, plants to be watered, and a yard to take care of. It meant a lot to us that the entire Spicer family in West Dover volunteered to take care of our house, including mowing the grass and weeding my first feeble attempt at gardening in a mountain climate. If the family lives in a city, managing their home from afar can be even more complicated and may require the services of someone to house-sit while they are away. Any way you can offer to help a family living away from home will be tremendously appreciated.

Someone to run errands or search out information. As a parent spending time with a hospitalized child, it is difficult to find the time and energy to run errands, wash clothes, go to the library, and so forth. It may not sound like a big deal, but one of the most useful gifts I got while Alex was in the hospital was a package of six new pairs of underwear from my mother.

Anything to alleviate the mountain of stress they are experiencing. Many gestures, great or small, are appreciated simply because they serve to reduce the tremendous amount of stress for parents. I remember getting a call from Suzanne, the special education coordinator of our local school system, offering to help coordinate outpatient therapy services for Alex. At that point, Alex was still struggling to live a day at a time, but I found comfort in her statement: Not only was she being optimistic, but she was also telling us not to worry about the future. I also remember when our parents sent us the money to stay in the hotel next door to Children's Hospital. It was like going on a vacation compared with bunking on a cot in communal sleeping rooms every night.

Someone to be the "runner" and "messenger" between family and friends. I don't think most people realize how utterly exhausting it is to talk on the phone for hours on end and repeat what is happening to your child again and again. Phone calls are perhaps the easiest way to say, "I care," but they can be emotionally taxing for parents. During the first weeks of Alex's illness, all the calls seemed to come at the wrong time and place. We wanted all of our family and friends to know how Alex was doing, but we didn't have the energy or time to call each one back. It was a great relief to us when Tom's brother and my mother offered to keep our extended family members abreast of Alex's condition.

If you can't decide what to do for the family of an ill or injured child, ask another family member for suggestions. And, if you can't add something positive to the situation, don't do anything. I can assure you that doing the "wrong" thing—something that inadvertently creates anger, stress, or guilt—will be remembered far longer than doing nothing at all.

Fifteen Suggestions for Things to Bring or Send

Alex received a lot of flowers and Mylar balloons when he was in the hospital. In the days before he could raise his head or talk, the balloons gave him something visually interesting to look at. And one of his first requests when he began to talk was to smell the daisy in the bouquet of flowers sitting next to his bed. These expressions of love from family and friends were enjoyed by all of us, not just Alex. Interestingly enough, though, I don't think most people realize that you can also easily send mail—letters as well as packages—and that they are delivered to the child's bedside, whether the child is in the ICU or a hospital room. If you want to bring or send something to the child or the family, consider things that entertain or provide physical comfort. And, don't forget that siblings may be visiting the hospital as well. Some suggestions are:

1. *Small or intricate objects to manipulate and observe.* If the child is young or is otherwise fairly immobilized by his or her condition, consider sending small objects that the child can manipulate or watch. For example, Alex was entertained for hours by some wind-up trains that we put on a cafeteria tray. We made bridges, tunnels, and other obstacles out of cardboard to challenge the wind-up toys.

2. *Dramatic play objects.* Doctor's kits, puppets, and dolls are excellent toys to cuddle and engage in imaginative (yet sedentary) play. A young child particularly has a need to act out what is going on for him or her in the hospital as a way of understanding it. A doll that is espe-

cially appropriate is a Raggedy Ann or Andy. It is a very flexible doll that can be bandaged, dressed, and doctored. In addition, it is an excellent modeling tool for pointing out parts of the body and for showing the child how to do certain exercises or movements.

3. *Toys that reduce stress or release tension.* Ill or injured children of all ages will appreciate quiet toys that can be played with independently and that can be used to release tension. These might include squeeze toys, pliable toys, and manipulable objects. Older children, for example, may use toys such as foam or Velcro dartboards to release tension. I've seen dartboards do wonders for the self-esteem of children who were able to challenge physicians, nurses, and other medical personnel. Remote control toys seem to be ideal toys for bedridden preschoolers and school-aged children because they give the child a sense of control while promoting dexterity.

4. *Books and tapes for the entire family.* I've always believed that a child can never have too many books. The many months we've spent in hospitals have certainly confirmed that belief! Parents also need books and magazines to pass the many hours they must sit and wait. Besides books, audio- or story tapes are great gifts—they have always been a favorite of Alex's. Of course, ask if the child has a tape player or if he or she can borrow one from the pediatric unit before sending tapes. Tapes the child can sing along with are especially good, since singing, and the breathing that accompanies it, relaxes the child and reduces muscle tension. Listening to music has also been shown to be an effective means of reducing pain in children by decreasing their anxiety and depression.

5. *Videos of family and friends.* A hospitalized child will enjoy some home videos or videos that you create with

family members and friends. Home videos are particularly nice ways for grandparents or distant relatives to send caring messages from afar. Or, you can check several children's books out from the library and make a video of you reading them. If the child is out of school for an extended period of time, you may also help the parents arrange to have some of the lessons videotaped. Videotapes are not as good as being in the classroom, but they can help the child remain connected to his or her schoolmates and the school. Bear in mind that home videos may be disturbing to toddlers who may not yet understand whether they are observing real interactions or a videotape.

6. *Personal care items.* Consider sending a basket of personal care items like scented soap, soaps in interesting shapes, fingernail clippers, emery boards, and tweezers. Personal care items beyond toothbrushes, toothpaste, combs, and brushes are hard to come by in hospitals. For girls, a manicure set, including some outrageous nail polish colors, can be both entertaining and a boost to self-esteem.

7. *Moisturizing products.* A tiny gift, but one that will be a favorite, is a tube of flavored lip balm or Chap Stick. The air in hospitals is dry—very dry. This is usually because hospitals have ultrafiltration systems to limit the transfer of airborne particles that spread diseases and contaminants. A combination of the dry air and the tendency to lick one's lips when anxious leaves every child's lips chapped and or cracked.

8. *Colorful scarfs, bandannas, and socks.* Children of all ages are conscious of how they look. Older children are aware of how others see them, and their looks have a significant effect on their self-image. Younger children are disturbed by any irregularities in their looks, particularly if

they involve restraint. Colorful material, scarfs, bandannas, or socks can be used to cover wound sites, hair loss, IVs, casts, and the like. During one hospitalization, Alex was concerned with the IV site on his arm. We made socks into puppets, cut finger holes, and placed them over his IV. It took his mind off the IV as well as entertained him.

9. *Novelty pillowcase.* Kids love novelty pillowcases with their favorite action figures or cartoon characters on them. Colorful pillowcases also brighten up an otherwise boring white bed. Alex has developed a whole collection of novelty pillowcases, and when he's feeling his worst, he imagines that Pooh Bear or the Lion King is taking care of him.

10. A *comfortable cup to sip from.* Ill and injured children often have to drink ample quantities of liquids. Hospitals readily supply straws, but it is difficult to get a spill-proof cup. A spill-proof cup is a very useful item to bring for children who are bedridden and unable to sit up or hold a conventional cup. It increases the child's feelings of independence and allows the child to control his or her liquid intake. For older children, a novelty mug or thermos can be a fun, useful, and inexpensive present to bring.

11. A *lap desk, clip-on book light, and felt-tip pens.* Even though modern hospital beds can be adjusted to many angles, it is still hard to write, draw, or do homework in bed. Children will always appreciate a small lap desk for use with these tasks or a small clip-on book light. Typically, hospital room lights are either harsh overhead fluorescent fixtures or dim night-lights insufficient to read by. Children will also find it easiest to write and draw with felt-tip pens. They take less strength and fine motor

control, which may be an issue if the child has an IV, is highly medicated, or is otherwise incapacitated.

12. *A diary or a journal to write in.* An older child may want to reflect on his or her feelings in private. Often older children find that writing and drawing give them a private means of venting feelings and a greater sense of control over what is happening to them.

13. *Art and writing supplies.* If the child can use his or her hands, art and writing supplies are always appreciated. They are a particularly good gift to give a sibling so that he or she may decorate the hospital room with artwork. The medical ICU at Children's Hospital in Boston encouraged artwork, and Marty made sure that Alex's was the most festive bed space of all.

14. *Hand-held video games or a laptop computer.* On the higher end of gifts are items like hand-held video games and laptop computers. Items like these are excellent healing tools for bedridden children. For example, the distraction provided by simple video games has been shown to significantly reduce a child's need for painkillers. A computer-literate bedridden child will appreciate a subscription to an on-line computer service/Internet connection that will allow him or her to communicate with friends by E-mail or make friends through bulletin boards.

15. *A beeper or a cellular phone.* If you really want to splurge, get the family a beeper or a cellular phone (or borrow one). A nurse in Children's Hospital lent us a beeper during the first few weeks of Alex's hospitalization. It made such a difference in our life because we were afraid to go outside the hospital for fear we could not be contacted in an emergency. In much the same way, a cellular phone allows the parents to be in constant contact

with the hospital (but it should be noted that many hospitals are prohibiting patients from using cellular phones *inside* the hospital because there is some concern that they might interfere with medical equipment). I would really have liked a cellular phone during the times when I was driving alone for hours on an interstate to and from the hospital.

After the Crisis Has Passed and During the Long Road to Recovery

We would never have imagined that coming home from the hospital would be anything but pure joy. But, after Alex's bout with the *E. coli* bug, we returned home feeling anxious and alienated from the world around us. We had grown accustomed to the medical support of all the hospital personnel. Without their assistance, we found it exhausting to be full-time nurses *and* run a household. We were afraid of minor infections and were frustrated by little things, like the ostomy bags that worked so well in the hospital and were an utter disaster for an active four-year-old. Much of the attention, concern, and support we had received when Alex was in the hospital was gone. In fact, many people reacted as though nothing had really happened. We felt so alone that we didn't think we'd ever adjust to the "real world" again. It is at this point that families with seriously ill or injured children can really use your help. Unless you've been there, I know it's hard to see that physical recovery and healing are not the same, but they are not. Alex came home alive and patched up, but it was just the beginning of our healing journey. What can you do to help speed up the healing process?

Don't judge the past or focus on the future. Parents whose children have recovered from serious illnesses or injuries need to talk about what happened, but they need to talk about it in an objective way.

They are probably still feeling a lot of guilt, even though it may not be rational—I know we were. Even the slightest comment, like, "You should have . . ." or "Why didn't you . . ." would instantly feed on our latent guilt and anger. We also found (and still find) it difficult to think about the future. We can't predict the future, and thinking and talking about it only makes us more anxious.

Offer to be there and listen. Perhaps the best thing you can do is offer to be there for the family and listen to what is going on for them. Long after Alex was home from the hospital, we still had to watch him twenty-four hours a day. The ladies of the Loose Knit Group, our church's auxiliary association, saw how difficult things were for us and offered to come into our home and cater a candle-light dinner for us while they watched Alex and Marty. It was a tremendous expression of love and caring.

Go slowly and allow the family to readjust to the aftermath of the illness. Families go through a lot of adjustments in the healing process. It is hard for them to listen to other parents talk proudly of their healthy children and their accomplishments without wondering, "Why didn't my life turn out the same way?" Parents go through a period of mourning, which is even more intense if their child develops a chronic medical problem, as Alex did. I still remember how it made me bristle when people told me how lucky we were. Tom says that it made him want to hit anyone who told us we were lucky. Today, I know we are fortunate that Alex is alive, but we didn't come to that conclusion without a lot of anger, guilt, and grief. As you provide comfort for a family that has experienced the serious illness or injury of their child, go slowly, reduce your expectations, and give them room to mourn their own loss without trying to compare them with anyone else.

Offer to help out in any way you can. The recovery period is truly exhausting for parents because the days and nights often blend together. You can offer to stay with the family and help cook or care for the recovering child and his or her siblings. You might also offer to accompany parents to support groups or offer to drive the child or siblings to medical appointments. During a period of recovery from one of Alex's hospitalizations, a friend offered to drive Marty the twenty-five-mile round trip to and from school. It was greatly appreciated, for it meant we didn't have to take Alex out in the cold and unnecessarily expose him to other children and winter-time viruses.

Offer financial support. If you would like to help out a family with a recovering child, but don't have the personal time to expend, you might consider offering some financial support. Financial support *after* a period of hospitalization is as welcome as during the hospi-talization. By this time, the bills are piling up, and the family may be feeling financially stressed.

15

HEALING THROUGH
THE INTERNET

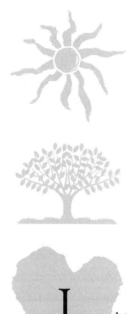

J ust as this book was coming to a
close, Tom and I were finally able to subscribe to an Internet
connection in southern Vermont at an affordable price. As writers,
we wanted to use the Internet as a research tool and as a means of
communicating with others around the world. I had heard there
were discussion groups for all kinds of topics on the Internet, so
when we got our Internet ID and configured our system, we
knew where we wanted to go first—we wanted to find a discussion-
based support group for epilepsy. We logged on, and Tom stumbled
through the UNIX commands to access the electronic discussion
groups (also known as newsgroups).

We requested a directory of worldwide newsgroups and then
searched alphabetically by category through nearly 12,000 listings—
through computer groups, science groups, miscellaneous groups, and

so on, until we found a long list of "alternate" groups. These are the newsgroups that are considered special interest groups, limited interest groups, or just weird groups. There in the list, along with other less serious newsgroups like *alt.alien.visitors*, was what we were looking for, the newsgroup *alt.support.epilepsy*.

The epilepsy support newsgroup, like most other electronic discussion groups, allows people to ask questions, answer questions, and share information with one another. You can respond either publicly, by posting a message or a reply, or privately, by sending a message to someone through electronic mail.

In the very first posting on the epilepsy newsgroup that night, a young man was describing the side effects of his antiseizure medications—the disorientation, the frustration, the confusion, and the emotional contortions he experienced. Tom and I stared at the computer screen in amazement. The medications this man was describing were the *same* ones Alex was taking. For the first time ever, we were able to attach a real-live person to the possible side effects listed so matter-of-factly in the drug inserts. As a five-year-old, Alex didn't have the words or the ability to articulate some of the sensations he felt. Often we had to guess what things felt like for him. It nearly made me cry when I matched the symptoms we read to what we saw and sensed in Alex. Tom shook his head and could only say, "Poor guy."

We paged down the newsgroup through many similar kinds of postings. There were informative messages and responses; compassionate, first-person accounts; and angry, frustrated ventings of feelings. Then we saw a question that caught our attention: "I know it sounds weird, but many of my seizures have occurred while I was eating. Does anyone know anything about eating and seizures?" For a long time, we had surmised that a trigger for Alex's seizures might be drinking a cold beverage when he was overheated. We had asked our neurologist about it, and he had told us that gustatory sensations could be associated with temporal lobe seizures—maybe there was a connection, maybe not. Here was someone else asking a similar question. We had been passively reading items posted on the epilepsy newsgroup for nearly a half hour, mesmerized by their contents. But, now we knew it was time to jump in and post our first reply. We composed a brief message relating our experiences with Alex and sent it over the Internet. It was midnight in Vermont, and Alex was sleeping peacefully in the next room, when we reached out to that guy in Australia to say, "You're not alone." I can't tell you what a magical moment it was for me when the server came back and said: "Message sent and copied." Goose bumps spread over my entire body. Had we turned off the light, I'm sure I would have glowed in the dark.

I was a teenager when Neil Armstrong landed on the moon. But I wasn't too young to recognize that I was witnessing a great leap of history in the making. As Tom and I sat in my office that night connected to the Internet, I felt for the second time in my life that I was a part of something that was going to change mankind significantly. It may be a while before people realize it, but I think Tom and I got our first glimpse of the extraordinary healing power of the Internet. We might as well have been back in the parents' waiting room at Children's Hospital commiserating with other parents. The intensity of the connection I felt to another human being halfway around the world was the same. As we read the messages, they were not faceless voices of an electronic discussion group to us, they were people struggling to cope with their family's illnesses just like we were. But what was truly astounding was the fact that they were there for me, in the middle of the night, in my own home, on my own terms.

The most remarkable thing Tom and I learned through Alex's illness was how to harness the tremendous healing power of other people. And, we learned firsthand that God's work is done through human hands. I sincerely believe that reaching out to other people and sharing information is a key ingredient of healing. In that respect, Internet support groups are going to advance our understanding of medicine in a way that biomedical technology cannot.

Our neurologist can describe Alex's symptoms and the likely progression of his illness, but he can't tell us *what it is going to be like to live with it.* That night on the Internet, Tom and I experienced a new dimension in our understanding of Alex's illness and the lifetime of healing ahead of us. For the first time outside the hospital environment, we felt *we were not alone—that there were others out there just like us. That night the circle of love extended around the globe.*

WHY INTERNET SUPPORT GROUPS ARE UNIQUE

At some point or another you may have attended a parent support group or may be considering joining one. All parents of ill or injured children I have ever met, including Tom and me, have needed desperately to talk to other parents who have endured the same experiences. Perhaps we find in other parents a truly sympathetic, nonjudgmental ear, or maybe only they can reduce our feelings of isolation. However, once you leave the hospital environment, parents with the same experiences as yours may be hard to find. Parent support groups can fill this need and may be excellent forums for working through your feelings and for obtaining useful information on caring for your child.

Unless you live in a major metropolitan area, it may be difficult to find a parent support group that matches your child's situation as well as your personal needs and time constraints. For example, I have always found it a catch-22 situation, trying to figure out how to care for Alex while attending a support group for helping me deal with Alex's illness. In addition, Alex's illness requires that either Tom or I be with him, so Tom and I could never attend a support group together. One of the principal ways in which an Internet support group is unique is that you can "bring" the support group into your own home at any time of the day or night. You don't have to drive anywhere, you can eat dinner while you "talk," and it can be as long or short a session as you want. There are many other reasons that an Internet support group is unique:

- You can silently read postings without getting involved in the discussion, or you can choose whom you want to respond to and whom you want to ignore.
- You can choose to be as personal or as anonymous as you want to be—all anyone knows is your E-mail address.
- You can be egocentric when you have a pressing question without having to worry about monopolizing the time of others.
- You can discuss very specific topics that may not be of interest to the group as a whole, and you may find many people who share the exact same problems.
- You have the luxury of taking all the time you want to think before responding to a question or comment—you are never put on the spot. You also have the opportunity to think about what you are saying as you compose your message.
- You can respond to the group, by posting a message, or only to a person, by sending electronic mail.
- You can access far more people with diverse experiences (e.g., people in other countries with different health care systems, different medical practices, etc.).

WHAT INTERNET SUPPORT GROUPS CAN DO FOR YOU

Internet support groups give you many of the same things you get from parent support groups, but in our case, we find them much more convenient and informative. Particularly if you are looking for information and knowledge as much as emotional support, Internet's bulletin boards may be just the medium for you. They allow you to learn about the latest advances in medical care, communicate with experts, and get thoughtful answers to highly technical questions because professionals as well as patients follow many of the electronic support groups. For example, we have found the epilepsy support group to be of great help in trying to understand the side effects of the many antiseizure medications on the market and their suitability for children.

About a year ago, when we were having a hard time controlling Alex's seizure disorder, our neurologist recommended that we try a new antiseizure medication. We had never heard of the drug, much less met anyone who was taking it. Our neurologist talked with representatives from the drug company as well as other neurologists to assess its appropriateness for Alex. We were all aware of its potential side effects in children, including anorexia, vomiting, insomnia, headache, and somnolence. In clinical trials with a total of 357 children, the manufacturer reported that there were statistically insignificant decreases in body weight. So we tried the drug for Alex, hoping that it would better control his seizures and have few side effects. After five weeks on the medication, Alex had lost nearly 25 percent of his body weight and was hospitalized, suffering from Stage 3 malnutrition. Clearly, it was not a drug for him, and the whole experience left us very skittish about trying any new antiseizure medications.

We've always wondered whether our experience with this medication was unique. One of the first things we did after discovering the Internet's epilepsy support group was to post an article describing Alex's side effects and ask others about their experiences. In the space of several days, we had about a dozen responses. A few people strongly believed that the drug was the best thing that ever happened for their seizure disorder, but most of them had stories similar to ours. One woman wrote about her daughter's experience: "She swelled, had a horrible body rash, was hyperactive, wouldn't eat, and began having mood swings." Another parent wrote:

"While on the drug, our fourteen-year-old son had terrible insomnia. He also became anorexic. The drug didn't even control his seizures very well. As soon as he went off the drug, his appetite returned and he slept regular hours."

Through the Internet support group, we got rapid responses from *real* people who had had *real* experiences with the drug. I wish we had known what we know now when we were watching Alex waste away to nothing on the drug. I think all of us would have agreed to discontinue the medication a lot sooner.

We are now facing the need to change Alex's antiseizure medications once again. Although his current medications are controlling major seizure activity, they appear to be increasing his distractibility and contributing to his short attention span. Basically, we have two medication choices: Depakote, which has been around for a while, and Lamotrigine, a new drug that looks promising. Before we agree to one drug or the other, we are going to listen to what other patients on the Internet support group have to say, adults as well as the parents of children with the disorder. This time we will have a far better understanding of what to look for, what Alex might be feeling, and when to discontinue a medication if it is not working for him.

The example I've used from our experiences is the epilepsy support group, but there are a number of other support group topics out there, and there are often several newsgroups for each chronic illness (as there are for epilepsy). More newsgroups are being added every day. Other support group topics you might find include

AIDS
Attention deficit and hyperactivity disorder (ADHD)
Autism
Autoimmune disorders
Cancer
Cerebral palsy
Cystic fibrosis

Diabetes

Down's syndrome

General children's health (including support for topics like
   breast-feeding, discipline, and behavioral management)

Multiple sclerosis

Polio

What Internet Support Groups Cannot Do for You

Internet support groups are no substitute for professional medical advice. *You should never interpret what you read on any electronic support group as a medical fact.* Rather, use the information you obtain from the Internet as the basis for a discussion with your pediatrician or family physician. For example, we will discuss the information we collect on Depakote and Lamotrigine with our neurologist in deciding what antiseizure medication to try next for Alex.

It is also important to note that *anyone can post information on the Internet support groups, including people who don't know what they are talking about.* Of course, this may be true in parent support groups as well. I think you need to read Internet support groups with the same healthy skepticism that you read everything else—even the newspaper!

Perhaps the greatest failing of Internet support groups is that they don't give you the immediacy of feedback or the shared emotions conveyed through compassionate hugs and other nonverbal means of comfort—words often can't express the depth of feelings and emotions involved in healing. This is not an insignificant limitation. But when I look at the feeling of empowerment that I derive from Internet support groups, I have to admit that I can be persuaded to overlook this shortcoming.

What Else Is Out There in Cyberspace to Help You Heal?

When it comes to the healing potential of the Internet, electronic support groups are just the beginning. There is a tremendous amount of supporting material out there to educate you, to help you take control of your child's illness or injury, or to assist you in understanding your rights as a parent of a child with special health needs. Within seconds or minutes you can go to various sites on the Internet or World Wide Web (WWW) and find all of the latest information you would ever want to read. For the most part, at each site on the Internet you will find menu systems arranged alphabetically by organization or topic. When you reach a topic of interest, for example, leukemia in children, you will often find many other references to other sites with more in-depth or related information. A sampling of the kinds of material you can access follows (the relevant Internet address is shown in italics):

- The latest research in any area of medicine. You can read about specific topics (e.g., seizure management at *http://synapse.uah.ualberta.ca/synapse*) or go to The Whole Health Page at *http://www.sils.umich.edu/~nscherer/health.html* for medical, health, dental, and psychological topics and access to the National Library of Medicine and the World Health Organization.
- Anything within the U.S. Department of Health and Human Services, including the Centers for Disease Control, the National Library of Medicine, and the Social Security Administration, at *http://www.os.dhhs.gov/*.

For example, you might use this source to gather information on your rights as a parent of a child with disabilities.

- Electronic discussion groups on alternative and holistic medicine (an example is *misc.health.alternative*).

- Information on various drugs, drug therapies, and drug interactions through PharmInfoNet, which allows you to search the database by either the drug's generic or trade name, at *http://pharminfo.com/drugdb/db_mnu.html*.

- Emotional support resources for parents experiencing bereavement (GriefNet, at *http://rivendell.org/*).

- Information on K–12 educational curricula, at *http://hub.terc.edu/edresources.html*.

- Newsgroups for school-aged children (e.g., *alt.kids.talk*).

A World Wide Web of Comfort

It gives me a great deal of strength and hope to know that there is a positive force out there like Internet support groups. I like the feeling of being connected to a World Wide Web of comfort. I like the fact that Internet support groups make universal goals out of sharing and caring. I like the sense of community they create, and the way they dissolve all cultural differences and geopolitical boundaries. After all, isn't this what healing is all about?

16

MANAGING
CAREERS
AND THE
EXPECTATIONS
OF OTHERS

When Tom and I first moved to Vermont to become full-time writers, we thought we had it made. We could go to work in our blue jeans, look out our windows and see pristine mountain ridges instead of a jungle of office buildings, and spend more time raising our children. And we really did have it made for a while, until the day Alex caught the "Jack in the Box" illness. What was a charmed life has become a psychological prison for us, since it is no longer a choice. Unlike a jack-in-the-box toy, we can't stuff our lives back in and start over. It's not that we don't like what we are doing or where we live. We love both of them, but our lifestyle doesn't hold the same allure for us that it once did. Alex's life-threatening seizure disorder has meant that living in the city and having successful corporate careers are no longer options for us. How could we watch him twenty-four hours a day? How could we manage his schooling and still provide for his safety? How could we get up in the middle of negotiating a multimillion-dollar deal and say, "Excuse me, I've got to go—my son is having a seizure and his life is in jeopardy"?

Today we are self-employed, as are so many of the parents of children with chronic medical problems and disabilities. We work in our home on computers hooked up to bigger computers. We have portable laptops so that our jobs can go anywhere we go, which offers us a great deal of flexibility in our workday and work life. Indeed, the information age has made it a lot easier for people like us to live in a remote area and feel connected to the rest of the world. With a telephone, a fax machine, and an on-line computer service, we can do library research, "talk" with experts, send documents, and post and respond to information on bulletin boards. Never a workday goes by, however, that Alex's condition is not on our minds and Alex is not within minutes of where we work. Right now, it has to be that way. Up until three years ago, our lives and careers were far different.

I remember the day I first realized that Alex and an investment banking career were going to be incompatible . . . and that was *before* Alex developed his long-term medical problem, actually before he was born. That day, I had flown from New York City to Chicago with my manager and our department head for a business meeting. We were sitting with our clients around a conference table next to a window overlooking the imposing but windowless U.S. Steel Building. I was the only woman at a table of four men, all dressed in dark business suits and starched white button-down-collared shirts. Smugly, I thought about how I was nearly twenty weeks pregnant and had managed to conceal it so far. I had put off announcing my pregnancy until it was obvious, for I feared reprisals from my mostly male, family-unfriendly colleagues, who would interpret it as "well, there's another woman who's not serious about her career." They believed that working all night and motherhood were incompatible. They were right, but I didn't think one should have to work all night to prove one was serious about his or her career.

The meeting dragged on and on, and the afternoon sun streamed in the window, making the room uncomfortably warm. All of a sudden, my stomach felt rumbly, as if I had eaten something at lunch that had not agreed with me. First there was one twitch, then another. I felt a whop, and it was then that I realized that I had just felt Alex's first karate kick. I wanted to get up and yell, "I just felt my baby kicking for the first time." It was a once-in-a-lifetime experience, and there I was trying to focus on a discussion of Chicago's commercial real estate market. Alex wasn't even born and I was already feeling the competing forces of motherhood and career pulling me in different directions. One of my colleagues in another department used to have her nanny bring her children into the office in the evening. She would say good night to them before continuing to work into the wee hours of the morning. I vowed I would never be that kind of mother. Oddly enough, Alex's medical condition has forced me to be true to my word.

Do What You Have to Do

Fortunately, most people do not have children with chronic medical problems. Most do not have to change their careers and lifestyles to accommodate the medical, social, and emotional needs of their children. But what happens when your child has a serious medical crisis? How do you balance the demands of your career with your need to be with your child who is seriously ill or injured? We've had that experience and can unequivocally say it's tough. It occurred when Alex was hospitalized after his first seizure at seventeen months of age. Tom asked for a week off to stay at the hospital with Alex, since I was eight-plus months pregnant. Tom's manager, who was not a parent herself, listened patiently. But she didn't ask about Alex, she didn't even say she was sorry, and she didn't offer to help in any way. She just coldly responded, "Do what you have to do." Six weeks later Tom's position was eliminated without any justification. Now he had a sick child and a newborn baby and was out of a job. Was it a cause-and-effect situation or only a coincidence? It's hard to say. His was the kind of workplace in which men didn't concern themselves with their families—their wives did. At the time, I don't think he realized he was being told, "Sure, take the time, but it is at your own risk."

Since then, Congress passed the Family and Medical Leave Act in 1993. It is a landmark law, unlike any other employee rights laws that have come before. It tells employers what they *shall* do rather than what they *shouldn't* do. For businesses of fifty or more employees, it provides for

- twelve weeks of unpaid, job-guaranteed leave for childbirth, adoption, or illness of employee or family member;
- employee benefits to be continued during the period of leave;
- employees to take the leave in blocks of hours, days, or weeks.

The problem with the law is that the notion of a family-oriented leave clashes with many corporate cultures. Those of us who dare to place our families above our careers, either by choice or necessity, are often selectively eliminated, as Tom discovered.

In many corporations, the law has been a failure. Employees report that they experience subtle retaliation after returning to work following a family leave. Their offices have been ransacked or their responsibilities on a major project have been shifted to someone else. Others need the leave but are afraid to take it because they fear they won't be taken seriously as an employee. Instead of taking the time to be with a sick or dying family member, they sit at work, ridden with guilt, and everyone loses. Still others find out that their jobs have been eliminated in their absence. My friend Muriel was one of those people.

Muriel took three months of unpaid family leave, and when she returned, she found her position as a real estate research analyst in an investment banking group had been eliminated. Under the terms of the law, she was guaranteed a comparable job, and she was given one in an entirely different area of the organization. Her title was the same, her salary was the same, but was the job really comparable? She had invested the past five years in the real estate industry, getting to know the ins and outs of the business and the key players. Forget all that, she was told, just start over in an entirely new business area. Would her job have been eliminated had she not taken the leave? Whenever you take a family leave, it is always an opportunity for your employer to see whether they can do without you. As Muriel's case illustrates, in the employer's mind, it's easy to demonstrate that they upheld the law. In the employee's mind, the law is a joke.

When your child is seriously injured or critically ill, you must make some difficult decisions concerning your career. On the one hand, you work because you need the money to live. On the other hand, you may have a child who needs you now more than ever. Do you "bite the hand that feeds you," so to speak, or do you place the welfare of your child above all else? Can you negotiate a position with your employer that will make everyone happy? Can you find support in the form of family or friends to share the responsibility you have to your child? Some of us are lucky to have flexible jobs or understanding managers. For others of us, the serious injury or illness of our children has a cost that goes well beyond the hospital bills and the emotional strain—it affects our livelihood as well.

MEDICAL CRISES AND CAREERS

What can you do to minimize the adverse effects of your child's illness on your career? Manage your career concerns with the same seriousness with which you manage your child's medical condition:

Know your rights. Once the immediate emergency has passed, never enter into a discussion of your need to take family leave until you are fully aware of your rights. If you work in a company of fifty or more employees, you are protected by the Family and Medical Leave Act. You can call your local legal aid office and ask for a copy of the law if you are unaware of its provisions. Many companies with a workforce of less than fifty employees have company policies to handle situations like yours. Read the company's policy, if there is one, before entering into any discussions. If your company does not have a policy, quietly ask around to see if you can find out how other employees were treated in similar situations. After researching your rights, don't be surprised if you know more about the law and company policy than your manager. You need not quote the law in support of your request, but simply be firm, knowing that company policy or the law supports you.

Explain your child's medical situation as honestly and clearly as you can. What little information you have, you should communicate as clearly as possible. This will give your manager a better idea of the reason for your request. It will also give your manager an insight into the degree of stress you may be experiencing and an idea of what he or she can and cannot expect from you. Often, your manager needs to communicate your request to a higher level of management, who may or may not be sympathetic to your situation. The information you provide will allow your manager to support your need for family leave.

Determine the amount of time you require. As best you can, try to estimate the amount of time you will be away from your job. Your employer will require this information in order to make plans to cover your job duties. If you are unsure of the duration, it is better to err on the long side, since it is harder for your employer to grant one extension after another than to plan around a single, longer period of leave. Employers don't like surprises—it puts them in a position of having to scramble around looking for coverage. Remember that even though you are in the midst of a personal crisis, *your employer still has a business to run.*

Try to negotiate a plan that will work for both you and your employer. Think of ways to suggest how you can fulfill your job duties without sacrificing the amount of time you spend with your child. For example, see if you can move your allotted vacation time forward. Or, if your job permits, try to arrange to work a nontraditional workday: maybe working nights, early morning hours, or weekends. For those parents whose work is computer based or can be done off-site, you may be able to arrange to work at home for a while. If you cannot find a way to satisfy your job responsibilities, you might suggest ideas for how colleagues or outside hired help (e.g., day workers, temps, or consultants) could cover your job. Your employer, who is not as close to your day-to-day job duties as you are, might find your suggestions of help.

Try to focus your energies on your work when on the job. Although it is hard to concentrate on much else when your child is seriously ill or injured, try to make the most of the little amount of work time you have. Minimize distractions at work by limiting the amount of time you discuss your situation with your coworkers and by screening all nonemergency or unnecessary phone calls related to your child.

If you sense resistance from your employer, document all conversations. Not all employers are understanding and accommodating. If you are uncomfortable with your manager's response to your request to take family leave, document every conversation. Keep a written record of the date, time, participants, and who said what in each conversation. You may need this information to defend your position at a later time if you find your request for family leave jeopardizes your job in any way.

Don't ever resign under pressure or in a dispute over the issue of family leave. If you work for a company of fifty or more employees, you are protected by the law. Even after the medical crisis passes, don't resign or allow yourself to be forced to resign if you feel you are being treated unfairly. That's often precisely what your employer wants. Try to work the situation out instead, for if you resign, you no longer have a defensible case. Besides, the last thing you want is to have to look for a new job when you are still reeling from the financial and emotional impact of your child's illness.

PEOPLE WORK FOR COMPANIES, BUT COMPANIES ARE NOT PEOPLE

A company may have a family-oriented, well-documented policy when it comes to family leave, but people are responsible for interpreting and enforcing it, not companies. Companies don't discriminate, people do. This is something important to remember if you need to take family leave. I once worked for a company that had one of the most outstanding records when it came to employee rights, but I had the misfortune of working for a department head who was motivated more by money and his success. For the most part, he operated within the confines of company policy and the law, but he engaged in insidious forms of bias that were difficult to prove. In a department of over fifty employees, there were only two women who had children—I was one of them. Both of us had managed to "slip through the cracks" by becoming pregnant *after* we were hired. Once he punished a male colleague who insisted on going home and joining his family for dinner several nights a week by assigning him to a dead-end deal in Eastern Europe for several months.

As far as this department head was concerned, requests for family leave were out of the question unless he didn't have a choice. He staunchly believed that there was no place in business for the family, and, frankly, a number of my colleagues supported his attitude. I remember one day how he told my immediate manager that he had to join him on a business trip to Chicago the next day to give a presentation. My manager protested that his wife, who had just given birth to their baby boy the day before, would be coming home from the hospital that afternoon. In so many words, he was told to make a choice between his career and his family. He went to Chicago and left his wife to take their newborn baby home in a taxicab.

I emphasize the distinction between company policies and the policies of the people that work for them because you need to be very clear on where both of them stand when you make a request for family leave. When you make your request, you need an ally who understands your situation and will safeguard your interests. If you don't find it in your immediate management, find someone in personnel who will be supportive of you. In the end, you do what you have to do, but you should also do your best to protect yourself.

The Real Costs of Having an Ill or Injured Child

Most people don't realize that they cost their employer more when they have a seriously ill or injured child. It's easy to take a benefit package for granted—you're insured if you ever have a medical calamity, and your employer pays all or a part of the cost. But, when you have an ill or injured child, your fringe benefits cost your employer more, and the demands of your child's medical condition leave you with less overall energy for your job. This is particularly true if you have a child like Alex, with chronic or recurrent medical problems. In the current cost-cutting environment, this fact alone can threaten your job. For a small company, your child's insurance coverage can be quite costly, possibly affecting the company's overall insurance premium rates. For larger companies, many of which have opted to use self-insurance for their employee benefit plans, your child's medical bills might be a direct cost.

Self-insurance means that instead of paying costly insurance premiums to major medical insurers, many companies are now paying out-of-pocket for a portion of their employees' medical expenses. They are betting that their employees will not get sick, and it will be less costly in the long run than paying large insurance premiums. When your child is seriously ill or hospitalized with a chronic medical condition, you cost more to employ, dollar for dollar, than someone without children or with healthy children. You do, however, have the law on your side: The Americans with Disabilities Act, which became effective in 1992, provides the same civil rights for disabled persons (including those with chronic illnesses) as it does for women and minorities. But, just as with the Family and Medical Leave Act, it is often impossible to prove that employers are not making an economic decision if they terminate you, or your job is eliminated due to the illness of your child. After all, it is always easy to argue that your work has suffered as a result of the stress you've been under and the time you've spent away from the job. If for any reason you suspect the cost of your child's medical problems are the reason for your termination rather than your job performance, make sure that you investigate your legal rights. A good place to start is with your local legal aid office.

Everyone Seems to Have Expectations

Managing the effects of your child's illness or injury on your career or job situation is no easy task. But, it is no less difficult to manage the expectations of others, including friends, family, and acquaintances. A lot of people will pass judgment on everything from the amount of time you spend with your child to your parenting skills. Some people will tell you to spend less time with your child—"Get a life," they say. Others will inadvertently make you feel guilty if you take some time off for yourself. I'm not sure whether people have a need to offer more opinions when you have a seriously ill or injured child or whether it just seems that way because you feel more sensitive and vulnerable.

Not long ago, I was sitting in a bagel restaurant with Alex and Marty in Brattleboro. It was lunchtime, and we had stopped for a bite to eat. Alex has never been a big eater, but eating has been particularly problematic since he acquired the bacterial infection. While recovering from his colostomy-reversal surgery, he developed a severe eating disorder that resembled anorexia and bulimia. Although we later discovered that much of his behavior was attributable to Felbatol, a new (and not well tested, as it turned out) antiseizure medication, he teetered on serious malnutrition for a period of nearly six months. His neurologist insisted Alex had to take in 1,800 calories a day in order to build muscle mass. But, Alex wanted nothing to do with food, and we had to practically force-feed him every meal. Even then, we could never get past 1,000 calories without him vomiting it all back up. For months after he was shifted to another antiseizure medication, we had to feed him because he refused to eat on his own.

Most of Alex's eating problems have resolved themselves, but he still requires 1,800 calories a day, and we still have to encourage him to eat. Often this means having to assist him in the process. That day in the bagel restaurant, he was excited about going to the city and was too distracted to eat. As we sat at the table, I broke his bagel and cream cheese into small bites and periodically popped a bite into his mouth when he refused to pick up the bagel and feed himself. At a table adjacent to ours, I saw a middle-aged woman and her companion watching me. She had a look of disgust on her face like, "What kind of mother are you that feeds a child of his age?" She even commented on my behavior to her companion. I felt the blood rise in my face, a combination of embarrassment and kindling rage.

It made me think about a scene out of my childhood when my brother, Martin, sustained a head injury in an automobile accident at age sixteen. His head had gone through the windshield of the car, and he had received nearly 100 stitches in his forehead. The Sunday morning after he got out of the hospital, we were sitting next to each other in church. My mother was sitting all the way down at the other end of the pew. Martin was wearing a piece of surgical stockinette over his mostly shaved head, and it was pulled down nearly to his eyebrows to protect his forehead wounds. In the middle of the service and without warning, a lady behind us tapped him on the shoulder. "Young man," she said in a schoolmarm voice, "don't you think you should take off your hat in church?"

I cringed. I already felt bad enough about what had happened to Martin and the fact that everyone was staring at him. I remember holding my breath to see what he was going to do. Martin calmly turned around and grinned a big toothy smile as he slid the stockinette up and displayed his still nasty-looking wounds. The woman gasped so loud that everyone near us turned around. She stammered how sorry she was. Normally, Martin and I would have cracked up laughing about a scene like that, but neither of us did. I've always admired Martin for how he handled that woman's comment—I knew it hurt him terribly inside, but he didn't cry, he didn't ignore the busybody, and he didn't get angry. He just confronted her nonverbally with the message, "How would you feel if your forehead were sliced up like this?"

Sitting in the bagel restaurant, I, too, could have done many things, from humiliatingly explaining Alex's medical history to the woman to simply ignoring her. I decided she didn't deserve an explanation, so I just looked over at her and smiled. But, I'd be lying if I said it didn't bother me. It's a scene that's repeated often, whenever I find someone "tsk-tsking" at me. It's taken me a long time to learn to bury my rage before it gets out of control. I just have to keep telling myself that other people's expectations have nothing to do with me and my family and the world in which we live.

If It Were My Child . . .

I don't know what it is about children that gives everyone the need to comment or offer their advice. It starts before birth with, "You should eat this or that," and continues from the first day of life through adolescence: "Shouldn't your baby be wearing socks?" "I wouldn't let *my* child walk to the store alone." But advice and comments truly become epidemic when your child is seriously ill or injured. I think of them as the "If it were my child . . ." comments, and they infuriate me. Several weeks into Alex's hospitalization for the *E. coli* infection, I went back to Vermont to attend to some business and spent the night. I was totally exhausted from the whole ordeal and went to sleep at 10:00 P.M., looking forward to a night of total darkness and silence. About 10:45, the phone rang and awoke me from a deep sleep. I answered the phone, terrified of what I might hear. On the other end was a well-meaning acquaintance who also happened to be a physician. He politely asked me how Alex was doing and then spent the next half hour talking at me, berating me for not searching for the cause of Alex's seizure disorder (as if it made any difference at that point).

"If it were my child," he said, "I would go to every neurologist in the country until I determined the cause." I learned long ago that it was worthless for me to argue with people like him. The annoying conversations were just twice as long. I also found that it doesn't work to cut people off and say, "But it's not your child," because you get the same argument just that much more vigorously. I found it was better to let people talk themselves out and then politely thank them for their advice. That night, as I lay in bed fuming, it was all I could do not to hang up on him. But I knew I would only be creating more stress for myself. Through trial and lots of error, I've learned that equal measures of stoicism and patience are the best antidote for people with expectations like his.

RECOVERY GOES ON AND ON

And then there are the people who expect Tom and me to be doing more to manage Alex's illness. In fact, Tom and I constantly have to ask ourselves when enough is enough. We could literally make a career of subjecting Alex to one invasive test after another to determine the true cause of his seizure disorder (although I'm sure our medical insurer would have something to say about it). We could also make a career of trying one experimental drug after another. But since we tried that with the new antiseizure drug, Felbatol, which almost killed him, we're leery of experimental drugs. Of course we would like an explanation and a cure, or at least a treatment that works for Alex.

It has taken us a long time to become confident that we wouldn't be doing anything differently from what we are already doing if we knew the cause of Alex's seizure disorder. But it never ceases to amaze us how many people expect us to commit our lives to solving the mystery of Alex's medical condition. We hear it from members of our families, from our friends, and from total strangers. Often, they refer to the characters played by Nick Nolte and Susan Sarandon in the movie *Lorenzo's Oil*, who would stop at nothing until they found a cure for their son's rare genetic disorder. Though the movie was based on a true story, it is still Hollywood, and who knows what it was really like for the parents portrayed? People with their own expectations for us often fail to see two things: that Alex is just one member of our family and that he is still medically and psychologically very fragile.

When Alex gets a minor cold, he becomes very paranoid and pleads with us not to take him to the hospital. We tell him to relax and that it is just a cold, but both of us know that "just a cold" has on a few occasions resulted in a hospitalization. Every time a new test, medical procedure, or medication is suggested by a specialist, we measure the benefits we would derive from the test against the medical and psychological risks to Alex. We discuss any of the tests or treatments recommended for Alex with his neurologist to make sure we understand them fully. If the objective of the test is simply informational—i.e., if we ultimately can't do anything with the results—we pass. We realize that there may come a time when Alex's seizures are so difficult to control that we don't have choices. But right now we do, and we always exercise them with our entire family's well-being in mind.

Managing the Expectations of Others

When it comes to managing the expectations of others, always keep in mind that you are your child's primary decision maker and your child's best advocate, no one else. No matter what happens, you will always be the parent of your child. Learning to deal with the expectations of others is another part of the healing process. It's not something that's written about in books, and, in fact, it's not often mentioned. But, managing the expectations of others takes time and consumes a great deal of your energy. For us, it has been an emotional journey of hurt, anger, awakening, and courage. Where do you begin?

Be confident about your abilities and your rights. Whether you are dealing with career issues or the expectations of others, focus on what you *can* do for your child. Investigate your rights and your child's rights when it comes to employment, schooling, services, and public access.

Think ahead about how you will describe your child's medical condition and how you will respond to advice. If your child has a medical condition, people will undoubtedly have something to say about it, and they may have expectations for you that you don't necessarily share. Think about how you will respond. Will you react emotionally, defensively, aggressively, matter-of-factly, or not at all? If you choose to talk about your child's medical condition in public, how will you describe it? Expect to receive lots of "well-meaning" but unsolicited advice. Think particularly about how you will respond to the unsolicited advice of family members without causing hard feelings. It is one of the biggest interpersonal challenges that families of children with medical conditions confront at one time or another.

Prepare yourself for the comments of others. I'm continually amazed at the things people can say and do. Think about how you will react to remarks about your child's appearance or behavior. Alex handled the last one himself, and I think he said it best. He was touring the elementary school with his preschool teacher when a sixth-grade girl walked up and said to the teacher, "Is he crazy?" (By now, everyone had heard that a child with a medical condition would be attending kindergarten next year.)

"No, he's special," the teacher answered.

The girl turned to Alex and responded, "Oh, you're special."

"I think you're special, too," Alex said, and gave her a great big hug.

It is difficult to anticipate all the comments people might make, but we try our best to be prepared for anything. By discussing how we have reacted to comments in the past, we try to put ourselves in a position of never having to think about what we *should* have done or what we *should* have said.

Think, "Family first." Maybe it is an old-fashioned value, but when we decided to have a family, we unconsciously agreed to place the well-being of our family above all else in our lives. But we didn't really realize it until after the fact—after Alex's medical problems came to rule our existence. It has taken us a long time to come to terms with Alex's illness and to be at peace with the decisions we have made: decisions about his care, his long-term treatment, our careers, and the welfare of our family. We have never regretted leaving our careers in business behind—they're pretty much a blur now. But we would always have regretted it had we not spent the time to become a part of Alex's healing process. We knew that we could always find other jobs even though they may not pay as well or offer the same rewards. But we could never have replaced the void Alex would have left in our lives. We talked Alex through a coma, we challenged him and his medical team to keep going despite the odds, and we are satisfied that we did the right thing. We've learned not to worry about the expectations of others anymore—it's our family, and our family comes first.

Epilogue

Just before Alex entered kindergarten, we moved to our new home in Marlboro, less than fifteen minutes from the hospital in Brattleboro. We left a lot of memories behind in our old house: good ones as well as bad ones. We'll always remember blowing bubbles on the grassy hillside in the summer and sledding down our long winding hill in the winter. But I hope we can someday forget the deck where Alex, suffering from malnutrition, broke his leg. And I'd love to block the memories of the room where the EMS people found Alex with blood trickling from his mouth and the pallor of death the morning he barely survived the *E. coli* bug. In the early summer months, salamander hunts have always been one of our boys' greatest joys. The eastern woodland newts we collected in and around the stream behind our old house have a life span of up to five years. I find it a little ironic that those tiny, defenseless creatures managed to outlast us.

After nearly three years, Alex is pretty much his old self. His seizure disorder is more or less stable for the moment. It's been nearly a year since he last was hospitalized, yet little neurological blips still plague him from time to time. In our new home, we finally got the courage to move him back to his own bedroom. By design, we located his room within easy earshot of ours. Alex started kindergarten in the fall, only a mile or so from our home. At the same time, Marty began his last year at preschool, showing everyone where to put their cups after snack and dazzling them by jumping off the top rung of the climbing frame. He is still, and probably always will be, healing from Alex's illness. Curly, our golden retriever, is a big dog now, and to this day, is still Alex's best friend.

And oh, yes, the cornstalk plant that Tom gave me for my twenty-first birthday—the one that we chopped down the day Alex was born. We moved it to the south-facing living room of our new house, where it sits in front of a two-story wall of windows, nearly eighteen feet tall. There we intend to let it grow and grow and grow.

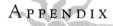

Appendix

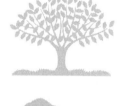

General Information for Parents of Ill or Injured Children
Association for the Care of Children's Health
7910 Woodmont Avenue, Suite 300
Bethesda, MD 20814
301-654-6549

This international organization of nurses, child life professionals, physicians, psychologists, parents, hospital administrators, and others is dedicated to promoting and protecting the health and well-being of children and their families. Excellent source of information, educational materials, and health-related bibliographies for both parents and children.

Center for Children with Chronic Illness and Disability
Division of General Pediatrics and Adolescent Health
University of Minnesota
420 Delaware Street
Minneapolis, MN 55455
612-626-4032

The center conducts research and training on issues related to the psychological and social well-being of children with chronic illnesses and disabilities. Publications include *Children's Health Issues* on recent research; *Children's Health Briefs* on single topics; and *Springboard*, a newsletter published three times a year.

Federation for Children with Special Needs
312 Stuart Street
Boston, MA 02116
617-482-2915

This is an education- and advocacy-oriented organization with a wealth of information on special education and coping strategies for parents of children with disabilities.

National Information Center for Children and Youth with Disabilities
P.O. Box 1492
Washington, DC 20013
800-695-0285

A federally funded project mandated by the Individuals with Disabilities Education Act. The center answers questions, matches families with common concerns, and maintains a database of information on national, state, and local organizations dedicated to serving the families of children with disabilities. The organization publishes *News Digest* three times a year and disseminates fact sheets and general information on disabilities to parents. A special series for parents, A *Parent's Guide*, is available at no cost.

Pediatric Projects, Inc.
P.O. Box 571555
Tarzana, CA 91357
800-947-0947

This international, nonprofit organization serves as an educational and advocacy group to promote the mental health of children in health care. It develops and distributes medically oriented books and toys for medically impaired and hospitalized children and publishes bibliographies on specific illnesses, disabilities, and medical treatments. The organization also provides information for parents on coping with their children's illnesses. A bimonthly newsletter, *Pediatric Mental Health*, is available by subscription. School administrators may obtain curriculum materials from Pediatric Projects, Inc., to assist them in teaching children to understand the disabilities and medical conditions of their classmates.

Illness-Specific 800 Phone Numbers

This is a list of toll-free phone numbers of national associations, advocacy groups, and information clearinghouses for a selected group of illnesses and diseases. Where available, organizations specific to the needs of children have been included. These organizations are an excellent place for parents to start researching issues related to their child's illness or injury. A more extensive directory of national information services on illnesses and disabilities can be found at the Internet address *gopher://val-dor.cc.buffalo.edu:70/11/.national.info/*.

American Burn Association	800-548-2876
American Diabetes Association, Inc.	800-232-3472

Asthma and Allergy Foundation of America	800-727-8462
Blind Children's Center	800-222-3566
The Candlelighters Childhood Cancer Foundation	800-366-2223
Children and Adults with ADD (CHADD)	800-233-4050
Children's Hospice International	800-242-4453
Cleft Palate Foundation	800-242-5338
Cystic Fibrosis Foundation	800-344-4823
Epilepsy Foundation of America	800-332-1000
The Feingold Association of the United States	800-321-3287
Lupus Foundation of America, Inc.	800-558-0121
National AIDS Information Clearinghouse	800-458-5231
National Association for Parents of the Visually Impaired	800-562-6265
National Association for Sickle Cell Disease, Inc.	800-421-8453
National Autism Hotline	304-525-8014
National Information Clearinghouse for Infants with Disabilities and Life-threatening Conditions	800-922-9234
National Spinal Cord Injury Association	800-962-9629
Spina Bifida Association of America	800-621-3141
United Cerebral Palsy Association, Inc.	800-872-5827

School Issues

ERIC Clearinghouse on Disabilities and Gifted Education
Council for Exceptional Children
1920 Association Drive
Reston, VA 22091
800-328-0272

The ERIC Clearinghouse provides teachers, other education profes-sionals, and parents with information on research, programs, evalua-tive methods, teacher training, and curricula for gifted children and children with disabilities. For a fee, you can conduct a computer search on the Exceptional Child Education Resources (ERIC) database and obtain various publications.

If you have specific questions or concerns about the impact of your child's illness or injury on his or her schooling, it is best to contact your local school district, your school nurse, or your district's special education coordinator.

Medical Assistance/Medicaid/SSI

Association of Maternal and Child Health Programs (AMCHP)
1350 Connecticut Avenue, NW, Suite 803
Washington, DC 20036
(for information on eligibility issues, state-specific programs)
202-775-0436

The Maternal and Child Health Bureau of the Health Resources and Services Administration provides financial grants to states for direct medical and related services for children with disabilities. Every state has its own plan. You can contact this organization for information on your child's eligibility for services as well as information on state-specific programs.

Maureen Mitchell
Children's SSI Coordinator
Parent to Parent of Vermont
1 Main Street, #69 Champlain Mill
Winooski, VT 05404
802-823-5256

Maureen Mitchell is a national advocate for children with disabilities and is an expert on SSI, Medicaid, and EPSDT (Early Periodic Screening Diagnosis and Treatment) programs. Although she is associated with Parent to Parent of Vermont, she has said she would be more than willing to help anyone who has a question about SSI, Medicaid, and EPSDT.

Social Security Administration
6401 Security Boulevard
Baltimore, MD 21235
800-772-1213

The Social Security Administration oversees a national program of contributory social insurance that pays benefits in the event of unemployment, retirement, or disablement. They can be reached through their toll-free number daily from 7:00 A.M. to 7:00 P.M. EST. Applications can be made over the phone, and recipients of their programs can obtain information on payments, payment history, and related information.

Your State Department of Health Division of Children with Special Health Needs:

You can inquire about available financial assistance programs in your state by contacting your state's Department of Health. Every state has a Division of Children with Special Health Needs. When inquiring, explain your child's situation and ask to speak with a representative about Title V programs.

Insurance Coverage and Disputes
National Association of Insurance Commissioners
444 N. Capitol Street, NW, Suite 701
Washington, DC 20001
202-624-7790

This organization can help you with situations in which you feel you or your family are not being treated fairly by your insurance carrier.

Legal Assistance

Your local legal aid office:

When you need legal assistance for a child with a serious illness or disability, call your local legal aid office first. Many states have programs that offer free legal assistance for disabled individuals. In the case of a Medicaid or SSI dispute, do not hesitate to seek legal counsel.

Bereavement

The Candlelighters Childhood Cancer Foundation
1901 Pennsylvania Avenue, NW, Suite 101
Washington, DC 20006
800-366-2223

This is a support organization for parents of children who have or have had cancer. Parent-to-parent support is available from the time of diagnosis through treatment, cure, or death. It is an excellent organization for bereavement support. Groups meet locally throughout the world.

The Compassionate Friends
P.O. Box 3696
Oak Brook, IL 60522-3696
708-990-0010

The Compassionate Friends is an international parent support group for bereavement with nearly 700 local chapters in the United States alone. Parents meet to support one another, tell their stories, and listen to the stories of other parents.

Siblings of Children with Medical Conditions

Sibling Information Network
A. J. Pappanikou Center

University Affiliated Program
1776 Ellington Road
South Windsor, CT 06074
203-344-7500

The Sibling Information Network is an organization of parents and professionals interested in siblings of children with illnesses, injuries, or disabilities. It serves as a clearinghouse for information on research and sibling support groups, and maintains bibliographies of children's literature on various disabilities and audiovisual materials.

The Sibling Support Project at Children's Hospital and Medical Center in Seattle
P.O. Box 5371, CL-09
Seattle, WA 93105
206-368-4911
E-mail: dmyer@chmc.org

The Sibling Support Project is a national network service that can connect you with the closest support project in your area.

National Parent Support Groups

National Parent-to-Parent Support and Information Systems, Inc.
P.O. Box 907
Blue Ridge, GA 30513
800-651-1151

Although there are parent-to-parent support groups in every state, National Parent-to-Parent Support and Information Systems, Inc., is a nonprofit, national database linking families with special health care needs or rare disorders. You can contact them directly if you want to network with other families for emotional support and information, or you can contact your local parent-to-parent organization. As best they can, parent-to-parent support groups try to match families of children with similar health care needs and disorders on a one-to-one basis. These organizations allow parents, who otherwise might never come into contact with one another, to share health care information and resources, and to support the emotional needs of one another. The national organization encourages families to join together to advocate for improved access to the health care system.

Selected Internet Addresses for Illness-Specific Discussion Groups

misc.health.alternative	Alternative health remedies
misc.health.arthritis	Arthritis
alt.support.asthma	Asthma
alt.support.attn-deficit	Attention deficit and hyper-activity disorder (ADHD)
bit.listserv.autism	Autism
bit.listserv.blindnws	Blindness
alt.support.cancer	Cancer
alt.support.cerebral-palsy	Cerebral Palsy
alt.support.crohns-colitis	Colitis
bit.listserv.deaf-l	Deafness
alt.support.diabetes.kids	Diabetes
bit.listserv.down-syn	Down's syndrome
alt.support.learning-disab	Dyslexia
alt.support.epilepsy	Epilepsy
bit.listserv.epilepsy	Epilepsy
misc.kids.health	Miscellaneous children's illnesses
alt.support.mult-sclerosis	Multiple sclerosis
alt.support.musc-dystrophy	Muscular dystrophy
alt.support.ostomy	Ostomy
alt.support.post-polio	Polio

k12.ed.special   Special education
alt.support.spina-bifida   Spina bifida
bit.listserv.tbi.support   Traumatic brain injury

Selected Internet Addresses for Health and Medical Information

sci.med.diseases.cancer   Cancer diagnosis, treatment and
                                  therapies
sci.med.immunology   Immune illnesses
sci.med.nursing   Nursing discussion
http://disability.com/cool.html#ch Disability Resources by Evan
                                  Kemp Associates, including
                                  The Parenting Resource Center
                                  Our Kids (Raising kids with spe-
                                  cial needs)
                                  Info on Children's Neurosurgical
                                  Illness
                                  Cognitive/Developmental/Learn-
                                  ing Disabilities
                                  Disability-Related Legal Re-
                                  sources
                                  Government Resources
                                  Links to Medicine and Health
                                  Resources
http://www.os.dhhs.gov/   U.S. Department of Health and
                                  Human Services
http://debra.dgbt.doc.ca:80/   HealthNET medical and health-
~mike/healthnet   related articles
http:www.yahoo.com.health   Information on health and dis-
                                  abilities
http:www.medical=web.com   The Medical Web: information
                                  for physicians, practitioners, and
                                  patients